Study Guide

Introduction to Clinical Pharmacology

Tenth edition

Constance G. Visovsky, PhD, RN, ACNP, FAAN
Professor
College of Nursing
University of South Florida
Tampa, Florida

Cheryl H. Zambroski, PhD, RN
Associate Professor
College of Nursing
University of South Florida
Tampa, Florida

Shirley Meier Hosler, RN, BSN, MSN
Adjunct Faculty
Santa Fe Community College
Santa Fe, New Mexico

Study Guide

Introduction to Clinical Pharmacology

Tenth edition

Denise Passmore, PhD

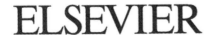

ELSEVIER

3251 Riverport Lane
St. Louis, Missouri 63043

Senior Content Strategist: Nancy O'Brien
Content Development Specialist: Sara Hardin
Publishing Service Manager: Deepthi Unni
Project Manager: Haritha Dharmarajan

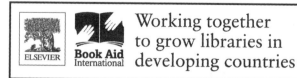
Printed in the United States of America

Last digit is the print number: 9   8   7   6   5   4   3   2   1

To the Student

The role of the LPN/LVN is becoming increasingly important in the healthcare system, particularly as many registered nurses retire and leave the profession. More and more LPN/LVNs will move into responsible positions in a wide variety of settings—both inside and outside the United States—where this book is used. LPN/LVNs must be prepared to practice in settings with advanced technology, many other healthcare workers, and increasingly complex patients, diseases, and treatments. They must also be prepared to care for patients in areas where they may be one of the only healthcare workers; where there is no technology; and many challenging patients, diseases, and treatments.

This textbook was written in a concise and simple manner to share important information about the complex process of giving medications. It was written deliberately to provide information that LPN/LVNs must know. The Study Guide is designed to help those students who are serious about doing well on the NCLEX exams and caring well for patients. The content has been selected based on what faculty from a variety of LPN/LVN programs agree is relevant and necessary.

Learning about pharmacology and the medications to give to your patients is important. Mastering difficult concepts and tasks is often a great source of personal happiness.

STUDY HINTS FOR ALL STUDENTS

Ask Questions!

There are no stupid questions. If you do not know something or are not sure, you need to find out. Other people may be wondering the same thing but may be too shy to ask. The answer could mean life or death to your patient. That is certainly more important than feeling embarrassed about asking a question.

Chapter Objectives

At the beginning of each chapter in the textbook are objectives that you should have mastered when you finish studying that chapter. Write these objectives in your notebook, leaving a blank space after each. Fill in the answers as you find them while reading the chapter. Review to make sure your answers are correct and complete. Use these answers when you study for tests. This should also be done for separate course objectives that your instructor has listed in your class syllabus.

Evolve Website

The Evolve website to accompany the *Introduction to Clinical Pharmacology* contains the following resources: Math review; Answer Keys to case studies, critical thinking questions and end-of-chapter NCLEX Review Questions; Drug Dosage Calculators; an audio and English/Spanish glossary; Interactive NCLEX Review Questions; Patient Teaching Handouts; and Videoclips. Using these resources as you study can help you master the material. The Evolve website for the textbook can be found at (http://evolve.elsevier.com/Visovsky/LPNpharmacology/).

Key Terms

At the beginning of each chapter in the textbook are key terms that you will encounter as you read the chapter. Text page number references are provided for easy reference and review, and the key terms are in color the first time they appear in the chapter. Phonetic pronunciations are provided for terms that you might find difficult to pronounce. The goal is to help the student reader with limited proficiency in English to develop a greater command of the pronunciation of scientific and nonscientific terminology in English. It is hoped that a more general competency in the understanding and use of medical and scientific language may result.

Key Points

Use the Key Points at the end of each chapter in the textbook to help with review for exams.

Reading Hints

When reading each chapter in the textbook, look at the subject headings to learn what each section is about. Read for the general meaning first. Then reread parts you did not understand. It may help to read those parts aloud. Carefully read the information given in each table and study each figure and its caption.

Concepts

While studying, put difficult concepts into your own words to see if you understand them. Check this understanding with another student or the instructor. Write these in your notebook.

Class Notes

When taking lecture notes in class, leave a large margin on the left side of each notebook page and write only on right-hand pages, leaving all left-hand pages blank. Look over your lecture notes soon after each class, while your memory is fresh. Fill in missing words, complete sentences and ideas, and underline key phrases, definitions, and concepts. At the top of each page, write the topic of that page. In the left margin, write the key word for that part of your notes. On the opposite left-hand page, write a summary or outline that combines material from both the textbook and the lecture. These can be your study notes for review.

Study Groups

Form a study group with other students so you can help each other. Practice speaking and reading aloud. Ask questions about material you are not sure about. Work together to find answers. Attempt to answer the textbook and syllabus objectives in your own words.

References for Improving Study Skills

Good study skills are essential for achieving your goals in nursing. Time management, efficient use of study time, and a consistent approach to studying are all beneficial. There are various study methods for reading a textbook and for taking class notes. Some methods that have proven helpful can be found in *Saunders Student Nurse Planner* by Susan deWit. This book contains helpful information on test taking and preparing for clinical experiences. It includes an example of a "time map" for planning study time and a blank form that you can use to formulate a personal time map.

ADDITIONAL STUDY HINTS FOR ESL/LEP (ENGLISH AS A SECOND-LANGUAGE/LIMITED ENGLISH PROFICIENCY) STUDENTS

First Language Buddy

ESL/LEP students should find a first-language buddy—another student who is a native speaker of English and is willing to answer questions about word meanings, pronunciations, and culture. Maybe your buddy would like to learn about your language and culture too. This could help in his or her nursing experience as well.

Vocabulary

If you find a nontechnical word you do not know (e.g., *drowsy*), try to guess its meaning from the sentence (e.g., *With electrolyte imbalance, the patient may feel fatigued and drowsy.*). If you are not sure of the meaning, or if it seems particularly important, look it up in the dictionary. (If you guessed that *drowsy* means something like sleepy, you were correct!). If there is a technical word you do not understand or remember, look for it in the index at the back of the textbook or in your medical dictionary. Write it in your notebook. Keep an alphabetical list of words you have difficulty remembering so you can look them up easily and review them before a test.

Vocabulary Notebook

Keep a small alphabetized notebook or address book in your pocket or purse. Write down new nontechnical words you read or hear along with their meanings and pronunciations. Write each word under its initial letter so you can find it easily, as in a dictionary. For words you do not know or for words that have a different meaning in nursing, write down how they sound and are used. Look up their meanings in a dictionary or ask your instructor or first-language buddy. Then write the different meanings or usages that you have found in your book, including the nursing meaning. Continue to add new words as you discover them. For example:

primary
- **of most importance; main:** *the primary problem or disease.*
- **the first one; elementary:** *primary school*

secondary
- **of less importance; resulting from another problem or disease:** *a secondary symptom.*
- **the second one:** *secondary school* (**in the United States, high school**)

Contents

Study Guide

Introduction to Clinical Pharmacology

Tenth edition

Constance G. Visovsky, PhD, RN, ACNP, FAAN
Professor
College of Nursing
University of South Florida
Tampa, Florida

Cheryl H. Zambroski, PhD, RN
Associate Professor
College of Nursing
University of South Florida
Tampa, Florida

Shirley Meier Hosler, RN, BSN, MSN
Adjunct Faculty
Santa Fe Community College
Santa Fe, New Mexico

1 Pharmacology and the Nursing Process in LPN Practice

Match the definition with the term. Not all terms will be used.

1. _____ A health-related reason for not giving a specific drug to a patient or a group of patients.

2. _____ The act of carrying out the planned interventions.

3. _____ A drug effect that is more severe than expected and has the potential to damage tissue or cause serious health problems. It may also be called adverse effect, toxic effect, or toxicity and usually requires an intervention by the prescriber.

4. _____ The intended action of the drug, also known as a drug's beneficial outcomes.

5. _____ The process of determining the right response by looking at what happens to the patient when the nursing care plan is put into action. It is an appraisal of the treatment effectiveness.

6. _____ Information used to reliably prove an individual is the person for whom the drug treatment was intended. Identifiers may be a person's full name, their medical record identification number, birth date, or even their telephone number.

7. _____ A name (or label) for the patient's disease or condition.

8. _____ A system to guide the nurse's work in a logical way. Consists of five major steps: 1) assessment; 2) diagnosis; 3) planning; 4) implementation; and 5) evaluation.

9. _____ A collection of information typically stored in a computer or electronic medical record.

10. _____ Reports of what the patient says he or she is feeling or thinks.

A. Adverse effect
B. Assessment
C. Contraindication
D. Database
E. Diagnosis
F. Evaluation
G. Healthcare setting
H. Implementation
I. Identifiers
J. Nine rights of drug administration
K. Nursing process
L. Objective data
M. Subjective data
N. Therapeutic effect

You are asked to see a patient who is complaining of gastrointestinal issues. Select the correct terms to follow the five major steps of the nursing process.

11. _____ As part of the medical plan, you analyze goals and write nursing care plans.

12. _____ The healthcare team labels the patient's condition.

13. _____ Collect complete information about the patient's history of illnesses and surgeries, including any drugs (prescriptions, over-the-counter, and herbs or supplements) the patient is currently taking.

14. _____ You administer the drugs to the patient following the plan identified by the healthcare team.

15. _____ You collect initial information that can be used as a baseline for comparison as care progresses.

16. _____ After administering the drugs, you assess the patient for any possible adverse reactions or more common side effects.

17. _____ The identification of the patient's condition helps you to teach the patient how to care for themselves.

18. _____ Assess the patient after administering the drugs in order to determine whether the patient's condition is improving.

A. Assessment
B. Diagnosis
C. Planning
D. Implementation
E. Evaluation

Identify whether each of the types of information listed are: A) Subjective or B) Objective data regarding the patient's health condition:

19. _____ The patient states that she is feeling nauseous.

20. _____ The patient has a temperature of 101 degrees.

21. _____ The patient's blood pressure is 140/88.

22. _____ The patient vomits.

23. _____ The patient describes the feeling of pressure in her chest.

24. _____ The patient weighs 150 pounds.

25. _____ The patient has an irregular heartbeat.

List three areas you should collect data about relating to the patient's drug history.

26. _____

27. _____

28. _____

29. When taking a patient history, which of the following are important drugs to list?
☐ Prescription drugs
☐ Birth control pills
☐ Skin cream
☐ Implanted birth control devices
☐ Makeup
☐ Vitamins
☐ Marijuana use
☐ Herbal supplements
☐ Tea or coffee
☐ Cocaine
☐ Aspirin
☐ Hair gel

Additional information that you will need to know to manage drug administration (fill in the blank):

30. _____ that include the name of the drug and the type of the reaction the patient experienced (in other words, whether it was a mild or severe effect).

31. _____ that may prohibit or limit use of some drugs (such as sickle cell disease, glucose-6-phosphate dehydrogenase deficiency, history of drug addiction, immune deficiencies)

Planning to give a drug involves four important steps. Match the process with each of the four steps:

32. _____ Know the major action of the drug

33. _____ Learn what the drug is supposed to do for the patient

34. _____ Learn whether the drug should be refrigerated

35. _____ What does the patient need to know to take the drug correctly?

36. _____ What does the patient need to know about potential side effects?

37. _____ Learn whether the drug should be refrigerated

38. _____ Learn the main drug interactions

39. _____ Learn the usual dosage, route, and frequency

1. Know the reason you are giving the patient the drug.
2. Learn specific information about the drug.
3. Plan for special storage or procedures, techniques, or equipment needs.
4. Develop a teaching plan for the patient

List one component of safe drug administration for each of the nine rights of administration.

40. How do you ensure that you identify the right patient?

_____

41. How do you ensure that are administering the right drug?

_____

42. How do you ensure that you are administering the drug at the right time?

_____

43. Who indicates the right dose of the drug you are administering?

_____

44. How do you know the right route to administer the drug?

_____

45. Why does the right reason matter when administering the drug?

_____

46. How do you make sure you provide the right documentation?

_____

47. What must you do after the drug administration to ensure that the patient has the right response?

_____

48. How do you manage the patient's right to refuse a particular administration of a drug?

_____

PRACTICE QUIZ

1. Which one of the factors listed below have increased the demand for LPNs/VNs?
   a. There are an increased number of people who request LPNs/VNs.
   b. There are an increased number of people who are living with chronic illnesses.
   c. There are an increased number of people who need home health care.
   d. There are an increased number of people who are on fixed incomes.

2. LPN/VN practice has shifted over the past decade. Although currently most graduates practice in long-term and community-based settings, where did LPNs/VNs most frequently practice previously?
   a. LPNs/VNs practiced mostly in acute care settings (hospital-based care).
   b. LPNs/VNs practiced mostly in healthcare clinics.
   c. LPNs/VNs practiced mostly in doctor's offices
   d. LPNs/VNs practiced mostly in schools

3. What percentage of a work week does a LPN/VN usually spend administering drugs to patients and monitoring their reactions?
   a. 40% of the work week
   b. 25% of the work week
   c. 5% of the work week
   d. 50% of the work week

4. The nursing process guides your work when administering drugs. What are the five steps that are included in the process?
   a. History, Monitoring, Administering, Charting, and Assessment
   b. Assessment, Diagnosis, Planning, Implementation, and Evaluation
   c. Planning, Documenting, Screening, Diagnosing, and Administering
   d. Assessment, Administering, Documenting, Planning, and Monitoring

5. Why is it important to do a patient's history when he or she enters the healthcare setting?
   a. You must determine if the patient is in the appropriate place.
   b. You will be able to assess the patient's ability to afford healthcare.
   c. You will provide the healthcare providers with information they need to identify physical signs of illness.
   d. You must diagnose the patient's illness before admitting the patient.

6. When doing a patient history, you will document objective and subjective data. Why is this important information to document on the patient?
   a. It can be used as a baseline for comparison of the patient's condition as care progresses.
   b. You can prove that you are completely knowledgeable of the patient's condition.
   c. You can tell whether the patient's information is accurate by comparing the objective to the subjective data.
   d. You are only responsible for monitoring subjective data.

7. Why is it important to ask what kinds of over-the-counter drugs a patient is taking?
   a. To ensure the patient continues taking them once he or she is admitted.
   b. To identify potential interactions with any drugs the healthcare provider may prescribe.
   c. To explain to the patient why taking over-the-counter drugs are not safe.
   d. To determine if the patient is reacting to an over-the-counter drug.

8. Although it is not your role to develop a medical or nursing diagnosis of the patient, what will you be responsible for?
   a. You will verify if the diagnosis is correct.
   b. You will not have any responsibilities once a diagnosis is made.
   c. You will decide how carefully the patient needs monitoring.
   d. You will decide when the drug must be administered.

9. After administering the drug, you notice the patient's condition has improved. What is this effect named?
   a. Expected side effect
   b. Placebo effect
   c. Favorable effect
   d. Therapeutic effect

10. Which of the following tasks will you do as part of your continuing assessment of the patient to evaluate the effectiveness of the drug you are administering?
    a. Taking the patient's blood pressure
    b. Questioning his family about any improvements they have noticed
    c. Reviewing the chart to ensure the RN is documenting any changes
    d. Determine if you think the drug prescribed was the appropriate choice

11. If your patient refuses her drug, what is the best response?
    a. Inform the patient that taking the drug is mandatory.
    b. Contact the prescribing healthcare provider and have the patient discuss with him or her.
    c. Find an online article for the patient to read.
    d. Explain the reason for the drug and answer any questions she has.

12. When documenting the administration of the drug, which of the following must you record in the patient's chart?
    a. The time the drug was supposed to be administered
    b. The time the patient requested the drug be administered
    c. The time the drug was administered
    d. The time the drug was left with the patient

13. What is the preferred route of drug administration?
    a. IV
    b. Intramuscular
    c. Oral
    d. Inhaler

14. Your 25-year-old female patient is given an antibiotic. What is one possible drug interaction that you should identify for this patient?
    a. You should ensure the patient is not using illegal drugs which would decrease the potency of the antibiotic.
    b. You should find out if the patient is using birth control pills and warn her that the antibiotic could interfere with the pill's effectiveness.
    c. You should find out if the patient drinks alcohol and warn her about possible interactions.
    d. You should find out if the patient will be adherent to taking the drug as ordered

15. Before administering the drug, you must read the label three times. Which of the following is NOT one of the times you need to read the label?
    a. Before you take the drug from the storage area
    b. Before preparing the prescribed dose of the drug
    c. Before opening the drug, at the bedside, when you give to the patient
    d. Before disposing of the packaging

2 Legal, Regulatory, and Ethical Aspects of Drug Administration

MATCHING

Match the term that is best associated with the situation described. Some situations may have two answers.

1. _____ Your patient refuses to take his medication, so you decide to crush his pills and mix them in his oatmeal. However, you must inform him or his family of your method of getting him to take his pills.

2. _____ Before you crush his pills, however, you refer to the Institute of Safe Medicine website to ensure the pill can be used in this way.

3. _____ You suspect that one of your colleagues is actually not providing his patient all the medication ordered for her pain. Instead, the nurse is using a portion of the drugs for his own personal use.

4. _____ The nurse who is taking the pain medication is violating the ANA Code of Ethics and is unable to fulfill his duties in a safe and effective manner.

5. _____ By utilizing these drugs for himself, this nurse has violated specific laws and may face fines or imprisonment.

6. _____ You must know the expected and adverse effects of drugs given to your patients and watch for signs that the drug is working the way it should. Knowledge of drug interactions is a critical part of safe nursing practice.

A. Do not crush list
B. Impaired nurse
C. Covert drug administration
D. Nurse Practice Act
E. Controlled substance
F. Drug diversion
G. Professional responsibility

CONTROLLED SUBSTANCES

7. Some drugs are identified as controlled substances because there is a greater potential for their abuse than most prescription drugs. Controlled substances are categorized I through V based on their potential for abuse. From the list below, identify the schedule designation (I, II, III, IV, or V) of each drug.

_____ Tylenol #4

_____ Heroin

_____ Fiorinal

_____ Lomotil

_____ Ritalin

_____ Lysergic acid diethylamide

_____ Ativan

_____ Percodan

_____ Valium

_____ Alpha-acetylmethadol

FILL IN THE BLANKS

8. As a LPN/LVN, you can dispense controlled substances only if permitted by your _____ board of nursing.

9. Scheduled drugs must be _____ at the end of every shift by the nurse to whom the agency has given the responsibility for controlled substances.

10. Dosages of controlled substances are dispensed by the pharmacy with an attached special _____ sheet on which the nurse must record the administration of the drug.

11. Drugs to be used for patients are kept either in a _____ cabinet or an automated dispensing system.

12. Access to these drugs are never given to _____ or any other unauthorized healthcare workers.

TRUE OR FALSE

13. Indicate with a T (true) or F (false) what information a legal prescription order must contain:

_____ the patient's initials		_____ dose
_____ prescriber's birthdate		_____ time prescription was ordered
_____ name of drug		_____ duration
_____ route of administration		_____ signature of pharmacist

MATCHING

Match the situation with the type of drug order that is applicable:

14. _____ A patient requires a daily dose of losartan for her blood pressure.

15. _____ A patient has an allergic reaction to a new drug that has just been administered for the first time.

16. _____ A patient is given nitroglycerin just before undergoing a cardiac CT scan.

17. _____ A patient is given Tylenol #3 whenever she complains of intermittent pain.

A. Emergency or stat drug order
B. As needed or "PRN" drug order
C. Single drug order
D. Standing drug order

CONTROLLED SUBTANCES

At the end of the shift, the controlled substance drug inventory does not account for all the dosages received for the shift. Below are three steps used to try and account for the differences. Fill in the correct terms to complete the blanks.

18. All _____ who have _____ to the key must be asked about drugs they have given.

19. _____ must be retraced to see if someone _____ to record the drug.

20. Patient _____ can also be checked to see if a drug was given that was not recorded on the _____ sheet.

21. If you believe there has been an error in the administration of any drug, list at least three steps you should take to ensure the patient's safety.

_____

_____

_____

PRACTICE QUIZ

1. As a nurse, you must learn about and follow three level of rules in administering medication. What are the three levels?
   a. International rules, federal rules, individual hospital or agency rules
   b. Federal rules, state rules, individual hospital or agency rules
   c. Federal rules, state rules, prescribers' rules
   d. State rules, individual hospital or agency rules, pharmacy rules

2. Federal laws define three categories of drugs, including controlled substances and prescription drugs. First, controlled substances; second, prescription drugs; and third … What is the third category?
   a. Over-the-counter drugs
   b. Antibiotic drugs
   c. Steroid drugs
   d. Illegal drugs

3. A patient who has been taking controlled substances for pain decides she no longer needs them. After a few days, she begins shaking and becomes confused. What is this condition referred to?
   a. Psychologic dependence on the controlled substance
   b. Lack of pain control due to withholding medications
   c. Method for gaining attention of healthcare provider
   d. Physical dependence resulting in drug withdrawal

4. Which of the following behaviors would lead you to suspect a co-worker may be diverting controlled substances for her own personal use?
   a. She is unusually pleasant during her shift.
   b. Her work ethic is not up to the institution's standard.
   c. She frequently reports dropping or spilling controlled substances.
   d. She is snacking more frequently during her shift.

5. One of your patients has just been prescribed a new medication by a specialist, and you are instructed to administer it. This patient has had a number of bad reactions to medications, so as part of your due diligence, what will you do to reduce the risk of an adverse reaction to the new drug?
   a. Ensure that the drug will not create an adverse reaction with any other drugs she is already taking.
   b. Administer the drug as prescribed as the physician would be aware of possible interactions.
   c. Avoid providing the drug until your nursing supervisor ensures it is safe.
   d. Crush the drug and mix it with her coffee in an attempt to reduce adverse reactions.

6. When entering the room of a patient who is under your care an at assisted living facility, you discover he is swallowing several doses of Tylenol. What should be your response?
   a. Report the incident immediately to his physician in case of adverse reactions.
   b. Remove the Tylenol and explain to the patient that he cannot take any medications, including over-the-counter drugs, without his legal prescriber's written permission.
   c. Distract the patient, then remove the bottle of Tylenol and dispose of it, based on your institution's policy for disposal of drugs.
   d. Contact the patient's family and inform them that he will not be permitted to remain on the premises if he continues to disobey the institution's policy on over-the-counter drugs.

7. You cannot administer a drug unless there is a prescription ordered by an individual who has prescription authority. Which of the following individuals would most likely NOT have authority to sign a prescription?
   a. Nurse practitioner
   b. Physician's assistant
   c. Psychologist
   d. Dentist

8. After moving halfway across the country to another state, you are ready to start work again, but have a few questions about what the state allows you as an LPN/LVN to do in regard to the administration of medications. You want to find out the Nurse Practice Act for your new home. Where would you find this information?
   a. National Council of State Boards of Nursing (NCSBN) website
   b. The official state website regarding licensing and renewal of licenses for all healthcare providers
   c. The state capitol library that houses all documents relating to healthcare practice
   d. Order a brochure from the ANA

9. Why does an electronic health record with the capability of scanning a patient's wristband provide more accuracy?
   a. You will avoid having to complete an inventory sheet.
   b. The responsibility is transferred to the nurse leader for your shift.
   c. You will avoid having to decipher illegible handwriting.
   d. There is no possibility of losing the patient's record.

10. Drug errors must commonly occur at which of the following points in drug administration?
    a. During drug preparation
    b. When bringing the drug to the patient
    c. At the time you give the drug to the patient
    d. All of the above
    e. A and C only

11. Almost everyone makes an error at some point in his or her career. Which of the following situations would make you more reluctant to report the error?
    a. You are afraid that people will think you are diverting the drug for your own use.
    b. Your license will be automatically suspended for an indefinite period.
    c. The agency where you are employed is unusually harsh and judgmental about drug errors.
    d. You are afraid you will be sued by the patient or his family.

12. What does the **black box warning** on the inset of the drug packaging designate?
    a. The drug is highly addictive and most patients will be at a higher risk for dependency.
    b. The drug has a higher-than-normal risk for causing serious and even life-threatening problems in addition to its positive benefits for some patients.
    c. The drug is experimental and unusual reactions may occur in many patients.
    d. The drug has been packaged in another country and may be contaminated.

13. Which of the following practices can cause you the most potential harm when caring for a patient with a communicable disease?
    a. Recapping a needle that you just used to inject the patient
    b. Touching any part of the patient without first donning gloves
    c. Removing soiled linens and not disposing of them properly
    d. Not wearing a mask at all times when you are in contact with the patient

14. The acronym "PINCH"—*P* for potassium; *I* for insulin, *N* for narcotics (opioids), *C* for cancer chemotherapy drugs, and *H* for heparin or any drug type that interferes with blood clotting—is helpful for identifying which category of drugs?
    a. Prescription drugs
    b. High-alert drugs
    c. Refrigerated drugs
    d. Specialized drugs

15. Why might you not be able to crush a particular drug and administer it to one of your patients who has difficulty swallowing the drug?
    a. Mixing the drug with food can generate toxins.
    b. The patient's family has expressly indicated that this method is unacceptable, as it will seem as if the patient's dignity is in question
    c. Crushing the drug will speed up the delivery to the patient's system, which may create adverse reactions,
    d. Your institution has a policy forbidding this type of medication administration.

KEY WORDS IN PHARMACOLOGY

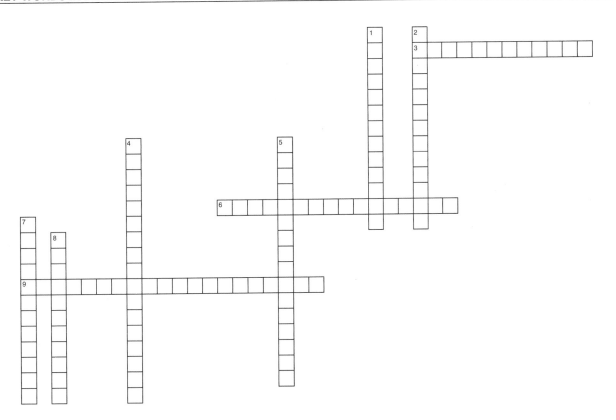

ACROSS

3. Drug that may replace another drug at a receptor site, decreasing the effect of the first drug
6. What the drug does to the body
9. The use of drugs in the treatment of disease

DOWN

1. Products that are chemically the same
2. Responses to a drug that are strange, unique, peculiar, or unpredicted
4. Process that happens mainly in the liver where there are enzymes that break down the chemicals that make up the drug into its usable and unusable parts
5. What the body does to the drug
7. Patients may see several specialists, each of whom may prescribe different drugs
8. These drugs have the potential to cause birth defects

Chapter **3** **Principles of Pharmacology**

MATCHING

Match the descriptions with the drug name. You may use an answer more than once.

10. _____ Drug name followed by the symbol ®, which indicates that the name is registered to a specific drug maker

11. _____ Most common name used for a drug

12. _____ Name used for a drug that is the same throughout the world

13. _____ Names that includes all the different substances used to make the drug

14. _____ The proprietary name of a drug

A. Generic name
B. Trade/brand name
C. Chemical name

FILL IN THE BLANK

15. Indicate whether the drug action described below identifies it as an agonist, partial agonist, or antagonist.
    A. In the case of an opiate overdose, naloxone is administered to a patient to reverse the effects of the opiate, which

    is bound to the opioid receptor sites. _____

    B. A patient is in severe pain and is administered morphine, which then activates the opioid receptors and produces

    pain relief. _____

    C. Buspirone is given to a patient who is already taking Prozac to help boost the effects of the antidepressant.

    _____

Fill in the blank for the following questions about how the body processes drugs.

16. The _____ process identifies how the drug enters the body and reaches the area it needs to affect.

17. Absorption of a drug is enabled through the processes of diffusion, _____, and osmosis.

18. Before a drug can enter the body's tissues, it must be dissolved in body fluid. How effectively a drug can dissolve is

    called _____.

19. Upon entering the body, the drug must reach site of action. The method of movement can occur by way of the blood

    or lymph system and is known as _____ of the drug.

20. Biotransformation is the process by which the body transforms the drug into usable or inactive components and

    happens primarily in the _____.

Fill in the blank for the following questions about the three mechanisms involved in absorption.

21. _____ is the tendency of the molecules of a substance (gas, liquid, or solid) to move through a semipermeable membrane from an area of high concentration to one of lower concentration.

22. _____ is the passage of a substance through a filter or through a material that prevents passage of certain molecules.

23. _____ is the diffusion of fluid through a semipermeable membrane; the flow is primarily from the thicker or more concentrated solution to the thinner or less concentrated solution

MULTIPLE SELECTION

24. Excretion is the process of removing the inactive chemicals, by products, and waste from the body. From the list below, check each of the methods by which chemicals are excreted.
    ☐ Feces
    ☐ Saliva
    ☐ Hair follicles
    ☐ Urine
    ☐ Bathing
    ☐ Sweating
    ☐ Crying
    ☐ Nail growth
    ☐ Weight loss

MATCHING

25. Indicate whether the following responses by a patient who has been administered one or more drugs are more likely to be (A) side effects, (B) adverse reactions, or (C) idiosyncratic responses.

    _____ Sleepiness

    _____ Stevens-Johnson syndrome

    _____ Liver damage

    _____ Nausea

    _____ Allergy or hypersensitivity

    _____ Bleeding

    _____ Diarrhea

    _____ Paradoxical response

    _____ Constipation

    _____ Kidney damage

SHORT ANSWER

26. Describe one drug therapy difference between African Americans and Caucasians.

27. Explain why individuals may require different dosages of the same drug.

28. Why do individuals with liver or kidney problems usually need smaller, less-frequent dosages?

29. How does body size affect the dosages prescribed for individuals?

Chapter **3** **Principles of Pharmacology**

MATCHING

It is important to identify the characteristics associated with the life stage of the patient. Match the characteristic with the life stage.

30. _____ Drug side effects are more severe

31. _____ Highest metabolism of all age groups

32. _____ Oral drugs poorly absorbed

33. _____ Growth spurts increase metabolism

34. _____ Higher percentage of total body water

35. _____ Dehydrates more easily

36. _____ Poor intramuscular absorption

37. _____ Hypotension

A. Older adults
B. Newborns/infants
C. Adolescents
D. Children

PRACTICE QUIZ

1. In order to avoid confusion over the various names given to drugs, many hospitals are now using which of the following drug names that is the most common name and is used in all countries?
   a. Trade name
   b. Generic name
   c. Chemical name
   d. Proprietary name

2. *Ethyl 1-methyl-4-phenylisonipecotate hydrochloride* is an example of which of the following drug names?
   a. Trade name
   b. Generic name
   c. Chemical name
   d. Proprietary name

3. For a drug to work inside the body, it needs to attach to which of the following areas in order to activate the chemical reaction between the drug and the body?
   a. Nerve cells
   b. Receptor sites
   c. Liver
   d. Mitochondria

4. Your patient is experiencing pain and it is not yet time for her next dose of pain reliever. What can you do to help her decrease the pain without the use of drugs?
   a. Massage her neck for several minutes to help her relax.
   b. Distract her with television or read to her.
   c. Get her to try simple yoga exercises in bed to help her stretch.
   d. Encourage her to do deep breathing to release the body's own endorphins.

5. Mr. B., a 78-year-old patient, is given a capsule to swallow, and you encourage him to drink a full cup of water with the pill. Why is this important?
   a. You suspect he is dehydrated, and the water will help the drug dissolve and begin working in the body more quickly.
   b. You are afraid that without enough water, Mr. B will choke on the capsule.
   c. The capsule has a strong taste that will be unpleasant to Mr. B and may make him reluctant to take his next dose.
   d. It is standard hospital policy that all patients consume a cup of water with oral drugs.

6. Mrs. X takes a Valium every night before sleeping; however, she has a difficult time waking in the morning. When you report this to her doctor, why does she replace the Valium with Ativan?
   a. The doctor suspects an adverse reaction to Valium
   b. Valium should not be used for more than 2 to 3 days
   c. Valium stays longer in the body because it builds up in fat cells
   d. The doctor suspects the patient may be becoming dependent on Valium

7. A patient in your care is being treated for high blood pressure. You note, however, that the drug is not as effective as expected, so you discuss it with your patient and discover the which of the following that indicates a need for increased dosage?
   a. The patient must take the drug twice a day and usually forgets the second dose.
   b. The patient is dehydrated, and the drug is not being distributed effectively.
   c. The patient has untreated sleep apnea and therefore needs additional medication.
   d. The patient did not report having liver disease and therefore the drug is not effectively delivered throughout the body.

8. Mr. Y reports having only one kidney due to a bad infection during childhood. Why is this important to know when monitoring his reaction to a new drug?
    a. Mr. Y may be prone to infections and therefore, it is important to identify any symptoms that indicate an infection may be developing.
    b. Mr. Y's decreased kidney function may indicate that the drug is not excreting effectively, and he may experience an overdose of the drug.
    c. The kidney loss may impact the ability of the body to dissolve the drug in a timely manner.
    d. Kidney damage is listed as a possible adverse reaction of the drug, so it is vital to ensure his kidney is functioning effectively.

9. A patient appears to be overdosed, but insists she only took the amount of long-acting drug as prescribed and followed all other instructions. Upon further questioning, you discover which of the following as the likely reason for her reaction?
    a. She experiences difficulty swallowing and therefore had crushed the tablet and eaten it with her morning bowl of oatmeal.
    b. She is overweight and the drug has built up in her fat cells.
    c. She usually takes the drug with an alcoholic beverage, which is contraindicated on the package.
    d. She has a slow metabolism and the drug stayed too long in her system.

10. Which of the following is a *paradoxical response* to a drug that should be monitored?
    a. The patient takes Benadryl and becomes drowsy.
    b. The patient takes an aspirin and her nose begins to bleed.
    c. The patient takes a steroid and his level of energy increases.
    d. The patient is on chemotherapy for breast cancer and feels nauseous.

11. Of all the factors listed below that can impact the safety and effectiveness of a drug, which one is most attributed to life-threatening adverse reactions?
    a. Drug-food interactions
    b. Drug-alcohol interactions
    c. Drug-tobacco interactions
    d. Drugs that interact adversely with other drugs, including over-the-counter drugs

12. Why is it important to note whether your patient is dehydrated or over hydrated when adjusting the dosage of a new prescription?
    a. Hydration impacts the blood flow, which determines how well the drug is distributed throughout the body.
    b. Proper hydration reduces the chance for adverse reactions to a drug.
    c. Some drugs react adversely to water.
    d. Hydration can impact metabolism, which controls the distribution of the drug to the liver.

13. What is one reason that it is important for you to know as much as possible about a drug before administering it to your patient?
    a. If you are not familiar with all the names, you may administer the incorrect drug.
    b. You will need to report at the end of your shift all the drugs you administered.
    c. You will need to know the most common side effects and observe for adverse reactions in each of your patients, particularly when giving a drug for the first time.
    d. You are legally required to identify all drugs by generic and chemical names before administering them to a patient.

14. One of your patients has just been given a new prescription; however, she explains to you that she is currently nursing her newborn. What is one way she can help reduce adversely impacting her baby with the drug?
    a. You can advise her to avoid taking the drug and try natural methods to reduce her symptoms.
    b. You assure her that the drug cannot be passed to the baby while she is nursing.
    c. You recommend she take the drug immediately after nursing so that it has a chance to be excreted before nursing time again.
    d. You suggest weaning the infant and moving to formula.

15. You have been instructed to give an intramuscular injection to a 5-year old child. To ensure rapid absorption, which of the following muscles is the best place to administer the injection?
    a. Gluteal
    b. Deltoid
    c. Vastus lateralis
    d. Rectus abdominis

4 Drug Calculation: Preparing and Giving Drugs

CALCULATION

1. Your patient has an order for 500 mg of amoxicillin. The pharmacy sends you 250 mg capsules. Using the dimensional analysis method, what is the correct number of capsules to give your patient?

2. The healthcare provider has ordered 2 g of amoxicillin oral suspension for your patient. The pharmacy sends you the drug with instructions stating that one teaspoon is equal to 250 mg. Using the fraction method, calculate how many teaspoons to do you administer to your patient?

3. You are to administer 40 mg of Lasix to your patient. You have received 8 mg tablets. Using the ratio and proportion method, how many tablets do you give your patient?

4. Your patient needs 80 mg of lisinopril. The pharmacy has provided you with 20 mg tablets. Using all three methods (dimensional analysis, fraction, ratio and proportion), how many tablets do you administer to your patient?

   Dimensional Analysis:

   Fraction:

   Ratio and Proportion:

5. What two types of insulin should never be mixed with any other insulin preparation?

   1) _____ and 2) _____

MATCHING

Match the definition or calculation with the appropriate intravenous administration term. You may use the term more than once

6. _____ How fast the IV infuses

7. _____ (Total drops to be infused/Flow rate) × 60 drops/hour

8. _____ Number of drops used to make a mL of IV fluid

9. _____ Drop factor × milliliters/minute = Flow rate (drops/minute)

10. _____ Differs by manufacturer

11. _____ Depends on the total number of drops, amount of fluid and the number of minutes the IV is to flow

A. Infusion time
B. Drop factor
C. Flow rate

IDENTIFICATION: MACRODRIP AND MACRODRIP

For each drop factor listed below, indicate whether the tubing that should be used is macrodrip (a) or microdrip (b).

12. _____ 10 drops/mL

13. _____ 15 drops/mL

14. _____ 20 drops/mL

15. _____ 60 drops/mL

16. _____ Used most often for children and elderly patients

17. _____ Used most often when faster infusion rates are needed

18. Amoxicillin, 500 mg, is a typical adult dosage. Using Clark's rule, what is the correct dosage for a 10-year-old boy who weighs 70 pounds?

17

MATCHING

Match the descriptions below with the appropriate term that identifies drug-types or administration routes. Use each term only once.

19. _____ Drugs given directly into the GI tract

20. _____ Drugs that must be shaken before administration

21. _____ Apply drugs to the skin or mucous membranes, e.g., topicals, patches, or ear drops

22. _____ Method used to inject between the skin and the muscle layer

23. _____ Has two compartments that contain a sterile solution and a drug powder separated by a rubber stopper

24. _____ This method seals the injection site and prevents leakage of the drug

25. _____ Method used to inject between the upper two layers of skin

26. _____ Drug administration that bypasses the mouth by use of a tube that goes through the nose and esophagus into the stomach

27. _____ Use this method when the drug ordered may be destroyed by gastric enzymes

28. _____ Method used to deposit deep into the muscle mass

A. Nasogastric tube
B. Parenteral route
C. Enteral drugs
D. Liquid-form oral drugs
E. Intramuscular route
F. Mix-O-Vial
G. Intradermal route
H. Subcutaneous route
I. Z-track technique
J. Percutaneous route

SAFETY CONSIDERATIONS

Answer the following questions about drug administration safety.

29. Before administering tablets or capsules, make sure the patient is able to do what?

30. To ensure a drug is evenly distributed throughout a liquid prior to administration, what must be done first?

31. Why is insulin considered a high-alert drug?

32. When a patient is unable to swallow a tablet or capsule, why must you check with the pharmacist prior to crushing tablets or breaking capsules?

33. What are some steps you can take to assist a patient who has difficulty swallowing the drug?

34. Why should you administer drugs separately through a NG or PEG tube?

35. When giving a drug subcutaneously, why should you avoid aspiration?

36. The preferred IM injection sites are deltoid, vastus lateralis, and ventrogluteal muscles; however, why is the dorsogluteal muscle *not* recommended?

37. When a patient is receiving intravenous drugs, what are some observations you should make to ensure the patient's safety?

38. When administering topical or transdermal drugs, why should you avoid touching the drugs with your bare hands or fingers?

PRACTICE QUIZ

1. Although many drugs are currently prepackaged at the correct dosage, what is at least one reason to know how to accurately calculate correct drug dosage?
   a. You need to ensure the pharmacy did not send you the incorrect dosage.
   b. The drug dosage ordered is not available in the pharmacy.
   c. Patients may ask you to ensure the dosage is correct.
   d. Some institutions require that you show calculations have been made before administering the drug.

2. How does The Joint Commission, a nonprofit agency that credentials and certifies healthcare organizations, currently recommend that all drug dosages for children be calculated?
   a. Weight-based
   b. Age-based
   c. Height-based
   d. Activity-based

3. What is a major disadvantage of administering IV drugs that enter the bloodstream directly?
   a. Patients may experience discomfort being attached to an IV.
   b. It requires more time in monitoring the patient.
   c. IV administration of a drug is often more complex and there is more possibility of an error in dosages.
   d. The potential for adverse events that range from allergic reactions to death is higher.

4. Which of the following is a basic guide for giving any type of drug to your patient?
   a. Always wash your hands before administering a drug to avoid contamination.
   b. You should always recap syringes after giving a patient an injection.
   c. Unwrap and remove drugs from containers before you are with the patient.
   d. If the patient is sleeping or otherwise engaged, leave the drug with the patient so they can take it at their convenience.

5. What is a disadvantage of administering oral drugs?
   a. Tablets resist the acidic pH of the stomach.
   b. Oral drugs are inconvenient.
   c. Oral drugs are more expensive than other types of drugs.
   d. Some oral drugs become ineffective when coming in contact with the acid and enzymes in the intestines.

6. How are drugs administered through a nasogastric tube (NG)?
   a. Tube going directly through the throat into the stomach
   b. Tube going through the nose and esophagus into the stomach
   c. Tube going directly through the abdomen wall into the stomach
   d. Tube going through the chest wall into the stomach

7. What is the best way to ensure the NG tube is most likely in the stomach?
   a. Auscultate over the stomach and listen for a 'whooshing' sound.
   b. The patient is able to take deep breaths.
   c. Test the pH of the stomach contents to ensure it is 0-5.
   d. Aspirate some stomach content and ensure you identify undigested food.

8. What is one common reason for administering drugs intravenously?
   a. Patient has a life-threatening infection
   b. Patient has allergic reaction to oral medications
   c. Patient is unconscious and not likely to object to IV placement
   d. Patient needs drug to act more slowly

9. Which of the following is true about syringes?
   a. Syringes are available in only one size.
   b. Calibrations are printed numbers on the barrel of the syringe and indicate the amount of drug
   c. The plunger is the portion of the syringe that holds the needle.
   d. The tip of the syringe is removed before administering an injection

10. When using a vial that contains parenteral drugs, what is one step you should use when filling a syringe with the solution?
    a. Air equal to solution amount is injected into the vial.
    b. The rubber diaphragm across the top of the glass container is sterile and should not be cleaned before inserting the needle.
    c. Do not remove the metal lid from the glass container.
    d. Insert the needle into the vial bevel down.

11. Which of the following types of containers requires a filter needle to draw up the drug?
    a. Mix-O-Vial
    b. Multiple dose vial
    c. Ampule
    d. Cartridge

12. Why are intradermal injections usually made in the inner forearm, scapular area, or the upper chest?
    a. These areas are less sensitive.
    b. The blood supply to this area is less.
    c. There is quicker absorption from the intradermal layer.
    d. The skin area has more hair and hides the injection site.

13. Where are subcutaneous injections given?
    a. Between the two upper areas of the skin
    b. Between the muscle layer and the fat layer
    c. Between the dermis of the skin and the muscle layer
    d. Between the lower areas of the skin

14. What is one of the primary reasons for giving drugs through the intramuscular route?
    a. Muscles are larger and therefore, cause less pain to the patient.
    b. You have more locations in order to rotate injections.
    c. It has slower drug absorption.
    d. It allows for more rapid drug absorption.

15. If aspiration is required for an intramuscular injection, what action do you take if blood is drawn into the syringe?
    a. Try again until you no longer withdraw blood then administer the dose.
    b. Discard the drug and syringe and prepare a new dose.
    c. Withdraw the needle and massage the area of injection.
    d. Wait several hours and try again.

16. Which of the following muscles is not a recommended site for intramuscular injections?
    a. Dorsogluteal
    b. Deltoid
    c. Vastus lateralis
    d. Ventrogluteal

5 Drugs for Bacterial Infections

IDENTIFYING TYPES OF DRUGS

Match the drug name with the category of drug(s). You may use categories more than once.

Drugs

1. _____ azithromycin
2. _____ amoxicillin
3. _____ doxycycline
4. _____ clindamycin
5. _____ ciprofloxacin
6. _____ streptomycin
7. _____ cefuroxime
8. _____ sulfamethoxazole/trimethoprim
9. _____ cefazolin
10. _____ linezolid
11. _____ imipenem
12. _____ erythromycin

Drug Categories

A. Penicillins
B. Cephalosporins
C. Carbapenems
D. Tetracyclines
E. Macrolides
F. Aminoglycosides
G. Miscellaneous protein synthesis inhibitors
H. Sulfonamides
I. Fluoroquinolones

SHORT ANSWER

13. List at least three disease-producing pathogens that can cause an infection.

14. Name two reasons why it is important for you to learn as much as possible about anti infective drugs.

15. Organisms are located throughout most of our bodies and are referred to as normal flora. What can happen when the normal flora is disrupted by antibiotic treatment?

16. When antibiotics are overused, or used incorrectly, what is the possible outcome?

17. The Center for Disease Control (CDC) identifies 18 drug-resistant threats in the U.S. Which three are considered urgent?

18. To improve the effectiveness of existing drugs, newer, more focused drugs are continually being developed. How are these newer drugs identified by healthcare professionals?

DRUG ACTIONS

Match the drug action with the category of drug(s).

Drug Action

19. _____ Interferes with the creation and repair of bacterial cell walls

20. _____ Prevents bacteria from making the final form of folic acid needed to metabolize

21. _____ Interferes with processes used by bacterium to make proteins needed for growth

22. _____ Inhibits cell wall synthesis

23. _____ Destroys bacteria by inhibiting enzymes needed for DNA synthesis and reproduction

Drug Categories

A. Penicillins
B. Cephalosporins
C. Carbapenems
D. Tetracyclines
E. Macrolides
F. Aminoglycosides
G. Sulfonamides
H. Fluoroquinolones

MULTIPLE CHOICE

For each of the drug types listed below, check all the statements that are applicable.

Penicillin

24. _____ Used for *prophylactic* treatment against bacterial endocarditis in patients with rheumatic or heart disease before dental procedures or surgery.

25. _____ The most common side effect is sinus congestion.

26. _____ Allergic reactions occur in 2–5% of the population, producing rash, *erythema* (redness or inflammation), *urticaria* (hives), *angioedema* (swelling of the skin and mucous membranes), *laryngeal edema* (swelling of the larynx), and *anaphylaxis* (shock).

Cephalosporins

27. _____ Used for uncomplicated skin and soft tissue infections, infections of the lower respiratory tract, central nervous system (CNS), genitourinary system, joints, and bones, and for serious infections, like bacteremia and septicemia.

28. _____ Nausea, vomiting, and diarrhea are frequent but usually mild.

29. _____ The most common adverse effect is tinnitus.

Vancomycin and Carbapenems

30. _____ Never used for infections caused by multidrug-resistant (MDR) bacteria in hospitalized patients.

31. _____ Side effects and adverse effects are severe, so use of these drugs is generally limited to young adults who are not immunocompromised.

32. _____ An unusual response is a deep red rash on the upper body known as "red man syndrome" that is produced by a histamine-released reaction.

Tetracyclines

33. _____ First-choice drugs in incidents of MRSA.

34. _____ Side effects include mild episodes of nausea, vomiting, and diarrhea.

35. _____ May cause permanent damage (skeletal retardation) to a developing fetus.

Macrolides

36. _____ Alternatives to penicillin for patients with a penicillin allergy and for infections caused by organisms that are resistant to penicillin.

37. _____ Most common side effects include mild abdominal pain, nausea, and flatulence.

38. _____ Can impair the liver and cause jaundice.

Aminoglycosides

39. _____ Treat serious aerobic gram-positive infections, including those caused by *Escherichia coli, Serratia, Proteus, Klebsiella*, and *Pseudomonas*.

40. _____ Intravenous administration can cause skin rashes.

41. _____ May damage the kidney (*nephrotoxic*) and can produce permanent damage to the inner ear (*ototoxic*), or hearing impairment.

Sulfonamides

42. _____ Used for treating acute and chronic urinary tract infections, particularly cystitis, pyelitis, and pyelonephritis.

43. _____ Side effects include *vertigo* (feeling of dizziness or spinning), *tinnitus* (ringing in the ears), hearing loss, and *stomatitis* (inflammation of the mouth).

44. _____ Can suppress bone marrow function, increasing the risk for anemia, bleeding, and reduced immunity.

Fluoroquinolones

45. _____ Effective against gram-negative pathogens.

46. _____ Common side effects are secondary infections.

47. _____ *Arthropathy* (joint pain and disease) can occur, especially in children.

FILL IN THE BLANKS

For the following general teaching information for anti microbial drugs, fill in the blank with the appropriate word(s).

48. Ordinary _____ is an expected side effect. However, excessive watery and bloody _____ with severe abdominal pain and fever is a complication and needs to be reported to the prescriber immediately.

49. If the patient develops a _____ in the throat, difficulty breathing, or swelling of the lips, tongue, or throat, call 911 immediately.

50. Instruct patients to take antimicrobial drugs exactly as _____ to prevent infection recurrence and drug resistance.

51. Instruct patients to stop taking the drug and notify the healthcare provider if a rash or hives develop while taking an antimicrobial drug. A drug _____ can develop at any time after the patient begins treatment.

52. Remind patients to report any new _____ that occur while taking antimicrobial therapy to the healthcare provider because they may represent an adverse reaction.

53. Tell patients that even though it may be inconvenient to take a drug in the middle of the night, it is important to space the drugs out _____ during the 24 hours for best results.

54. Instruct patients not to save antimicrobial drugs because many out-of-date drugs _____ and become less effective.

23

1. Mrs. Jones fell while gardening, causing a deep scrape in her leg. After a few days, she noted the scraped area was becoming swollen and dark red. She presents at the clinic and you immediately note the area is becoming infected. The healthcare provider confirms your suspicions and prescribes antibiotics. Before Mrs. Jones leaves, you want to ensure she does not develop a secondary yeast infection. In addition to probiotic capsules, what are some dietary recommendations you can make to Mrs. Jones to help prevent yeast infections? (Select all that apply.)
   1. Yogurt
   2. Dark chocolate
   3. Bananas
   4. Miso soup
   5. Beef
   6. Pickles
   7. Sauerkraut
   8. Eggs

2. Mrs. Smith's healthcare provider is preparing her for a regimen of antimicrobial drug therapy. You are going to assess Mrs. Smith to ensure safety. Which of the following actions do you need to perform in an assessment of Mrs. Smith? (Select all that apply.)
   1. Take a drug history from Mrs. Smith to ensure there are no drug interactions.
   2. Focus on assessing the current condition of the infectious site.
   3. Take vital signs.
   4. Assess how often Mrs. Smith bathes and cleans the infected area
   5. If ordered, get specimens for culture and drug sensitivity.
   6. Ask about any specific drug allergies.
   7. Prepare for allergic reactions.
   8. If Mrs. Smith is taking oral contraceptives, inform her that she may need an alternative method of birth control.
   9. Find out if Mrs. Smith has any religious issues with taking antibiotics.

PRACTICE QUIZ

1. Which of the following descriptions best identifies infections?
   a. An over production of the body's normal flora that upsets the pH balance of the tissue.
   b. Invasion of tissue by disease-producing pathogens that multiply and produce toxins.
   c. Invasion of the body of parasitical bacteria that disrupts the ability of the body to produce antibodies.
   d. Disruption of the body's existing microbiome, which invades the tissue and organs.

2. How do antibiotics impact the normal flora of the body?
   a. Antibiotic use strengthens the normal flora balance in the body.
   b. Normal flora of the body can impact the ability of antibiotics to destroy or weaken bacterial infections.
   c. Normal flora protect the body from damage by antibiotics.
   d. Antibiotics can kill off the normal flora, causing yeast or fungal infections.

3. Why are gram-negative bacteria more difficult to treat than gram-positive bacteria?
   a. The cell wall is more complex, with an outer capsule and two cell wall membranes.
   b. Gram-positive bacteria have a thin cell wall and no outer capsule.
   c. Gram-negative bacteria have developed resistance to most first generation antibiotics.
   d. Gram-positive bacteria have poorly formed cellular structures.

4. Which of the following organisms is a common human parasite?
   a. Mycosis
   b. Nectotrophs
   c. Helminthes
   d. *Streptococcus viridans*

5. What is a superbug or a multidrug-resistant (MDR) organism?
   a. An organism resistant to three or more different types of antibiotic drugs
   b. An organism that is resistant to all antibiotic drugs and is usually treated through chemotherapy or surgery
   c. An organism that is resistant to penicillin.
   d. Drug-resistant bacteria spread by birds and animals.

6. If a female is taking oral contraceptives, what should you advise her to do if an antibiotic drug is prescribed?
   a. Review optional types of antibiotics with her prescriber that won't interfere with her contraceptive.
   b. Use another form of birth control during treatment to avoid conception.
   c. Advise her to avoid sexual relations during drug therapy to prevent infecting her partner.
   d. Assure her that antibiotics do not affect other drugs she may be currently taking, including oral contraceptives.

7. When taking strong antibiotics, patients could develop pseudomembranous colitis. What organism is responsible for this condition?
   a. *E. coli*
   b. *Helicobacter pylori*
   c. *Mycoplasma pneumoniae*
   d. *Clostridium difficile*

8. Why should you always be aware of the start and stop dates of antimicrobial drugs such as aminoglycoside antibiotics?
   a. Excessive exposure can create adverse effects that permanently damage the patient's health.
   b. Excessive exposure can reduce effectiveness and increase chances the infection will return.
   c. Excessive exposure to antimicrobial drugs can create sterility in both men and women.
   d. Excessive exposure can increase the chances that the patient will develop an allergic reaction.

9. A major nursing responsibility with antimicrobial therapy is evaluating the effectiveness of the drug prescribed for the infection. Which of the following actions are necessary for evaluation of the patient's response to the antimicrobial therapy?
   a. It is important to know what the typical symptoms of most bacterial infections are to determine if the patient is actually infected.
   b. Symptoms should improve 5 to 7 days after beginning drug therapy.
   c. Ensure the patient takes all the drug as prescribed unless symptoms improve within 72 hours.
   d. Review laboratory work to ensure there are no adverse effects to the liver or kidneys.

10. Which of the following is NOT part of the assessment for antimicrobial therapy?
   a. Take a complete drug history from the patient to prevent possible drug interactions.
   b. If ordered, obtain specimens for culture and sensitivity before starting antibiotic therapy to ensure drug sensitivity.
   c. If symptoms continue at the same intensity beyond 72 hours or become worse, notify the prescriber.*
   d. Have emergency drugs and equipment available to treat allergic and/or anaphylaxis (diphenhydramine, epinephrine, crash cart).

6 Drugs for Tuberculosis, Fungal, and Parasitic Infections

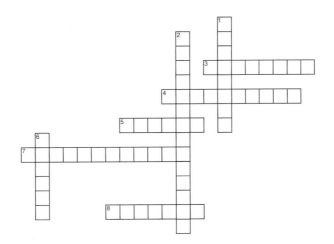

ACROSS

3. Microscopic, living organisms that exist everywhere and are both beneficial and dangerous
4. Parasitic worms
5. The most common adverse effect from antifungal drugs
7. A common lung infection cause by a slow-growing aerobic bacterium
8. A fungal infection

DOWN

1. An organism that lives on or in a human and relies on the human for its food and other functions
2. Drugs with mechanisms of action that only suppress or slow bacterial growth
6. A group of microorganisms that are everywhere and exist by absorbing nutrients from a host organism

DRUG CATEGORIZATION

Match the drug name with the category of drugs.

Drugs

9. _____ nystatin

10. _____ pyrazinamide

11. _____ fluconazole

12. _____ iodoquinol

13. _____ ethambutol

14. _____ praziquantel

15. _____ rifampin

16. _____ isoniazid

17. _____ metronidazole

18. _____ chloroquine

Drug Categories

A. First-line drug therapies for tuberculosis
B. Common antifungal drugs
C. Common antiparasitic drugs
D. Anthelmintics

19. List at least three symptoms of a tuberculosis (TB) infection.

20. How long does the initial phase for TB therapy last?

21. What are the three first-line drugs prescribed for children who have active TB or who are heavily exposed and require prophylaxis?

22. During implementation of TB therapy, what are the symptoms to monitor that may indicate liver toxicity?

23. What is the suffix for the drugs that are fungicidal and fungistatic?

24. How does Stevens-Johnson syndrome present in patients having this rare adverse reaction to antifungal drugs?

25. What are the three main classes of parasites that can cause disease in humans?

MULTIPLE CHOICE

For each of the drug types listed below, check all the statements that are applicable.

Antitubercular Drugs

26. _____ Used to control the active disease and prevent its spread to various organ systems in the infected patient or to other people

27. _____ Side effects include nausea, vomiting, diarrhea, headache, and sleeplessness

28. _____ Causes cardiovascular incidents

Antifungal Drugs

29. _____ Used orally, intravenously, topically, and vaginally to treat a variety of viral infections

30. _____ Nausea, vomiting, and diarrhea are the most common expected side effects.

31. _____ Adverse reactions are associated with more severe problems such as toxicity to the neurological, cardiac, hematologic, liver, and renal systems.

Antiparasitic Drugs

32. _____ Inhibits DNA and RNA enzymes and decreases the pH inside the parasite so it is able to use the hemoglobin in the human RBC

33. _____ May cause nosebleed and depression

34. _____ Optic neuritis can occur with symptoms of eye pain or vision changes, and permanent vision loss can occur.

Anthelmintics

35. _____ Used in destroying worms that enter the body, usually through contaminated water or food.

36. _____ Nausea, vomiting, headache, abdominal pain, and drowsiness are common side effects.

37. _____ Praziquantel can worsen symptoms of arthritis.

FILL IN THE BLANKS

For the following general teaching information for antitubercular, antiparasitic, and antifungal drugs, fill in the blank with the appropriate word(s)

38. Do not drink _____ for the entire duration of your TB treatment because all of these drugs can damage your liver and the damage is worse when _____ is consumed.

39. When taking more than one capsule per dose of antifungal medicine, taking one capsule every _____ or more can reduce the likelihood of GI upset.

40. Take antiparasitics with a _____ to prevent stomach upset.

41. Anthelmintic therapy usually involves an initial treatment that should kill all _____, but in some cases, a second course must be taken.

42. Do not wear _____ while taking the combination drugs for TB because rifampin can permanently stain them.

43. Notify your healthcare provider if you have dark _____, light-colored _____, or yellowing of the _____ while taking antifungal drugs because these are signs of liver problems.

44. When traveling to areas where _____ is common, take prophylactic doses of antiparasitics as prescribed.

45. You may need _____ supplements and an _____ diet to counteract anemia during hookworm treatment.

CASE STUDY

Elaine Benton is a 56-year-old woman who was diagnosed with diabetes when she was a child. She presents with peeling, blistering, itching, burning, and redness of the skin on her arms, feet, legs, and face. You think based on the condition of her skin it is a fungal infection. Because her immune system is weakened from diabetes, the fungal infection appears to have become systemic. After confirming the diagnosis with the healthcare provider, a prescription is given for the antifungal drug flucytosine. Elaine takes the drug for several weeks with some improvement of her fungal infections. She returns to the clinic for a follow-up appointment and you find she has a urinary tract infection.

1. In addition to a weakened immune system from the diabetes, why might Elaine be more susceptible to opportunistic infections? (Choose the correct answer)
   1. Elaine was not given the antifungal drug intravenously, which would have prevented the opportunistic infection.
   2. A premedication, such as a corticosteroid or antihistamine, was not administered to Elaine before starting the antifungal drug in order to avoid infections.
   3. Flucytosine can decrease Elaine's WBC, therefore increasing her risk for infection.
   4. Elaine is prone to UTIs and you anticipated this response.

2. What should be closely monitored while Elaine is taking flucytosine?
   1. Increase in hair loss
   2. Hematologic, renal, and hepatic status
   3. Cardiac dysrhythmias
   4. Glucose levels

PRACTICE QUIZ

1. What is the general cause of superinfections?
   a. The use of amphotericin B
   b. TB therapy that requires six months of antimicrobial treatment
   c. Antifungals given together with corticosteroid therapy, which reduces the immunity response
   d. Infections that are resistant to the majority of antibiotics currently on the market

2. After the initial phase of TB therapy, a continuation phase follows that lasts for how long?
   a. 6 months
   b. 7 weeks
   c. 1 year
   d. 18 weeks

3. How does isoniazid (INH) work against TB?
   a. Inhibits a TB enzyme needed for making its DNA and proteins
   b. Inhibits the enzymes of the TB organisms needed for reproduction and growth
   c. Makes the pH of infected cells lower (more acidic)
   d. Interferes with the RNA and protein synthesis of the TB organism, which reduces bacterial reproduction

4. How do azoles, polyenes, and allylamines treat fungal and mycotic infections?
   a. Prevents the production of a lipid-like substance from forming the fungal cell membrane, which damages the cell and it either dies or cannot reproduce
   b. Disrupts the metabolic pathway of the fungal cell
   c. Damages the cell wall and therefore kills it
   d. Stops reproduction and growth of the cell

5. What can azoles given at high doses cause?
   a. Increased sensitivity to the sun
   b. Numbness and tingling of fingers
   c. Reduced white blood count, which increases the risk of infection
   d. Life-threatening cardiac dysrhythmias

6. How do patients contract the protozoans amoebiasis and giardiasis?
   a. Mosquito bites
   b. Food and water contaminated by feces or by unwashed hands after using the bathroom or changing a diaper
   c. Handling contaminated soil, cat litter, and raw meat and then touching the mouth, nose, or eyes
   d. Sexual exposure

7. What is the drug albendazole (Albenza) routinely used to treat?
   a. Malaria
   b. Flukes
   c. Tapeworms, roundworms and flatworms
   d. Pinworms

8. What are the symptoms of trichomoniasis?
   a. Burning, itching, redness, and vaginal or penile discharge
   b. Diarrhea, abdominal pain, vomiting, and foul-smelling stools
   c. Liver abscesses
   d. Anemia

9. If your patient is hospitalized for tuberculosis and cannot take oral drugs, what other form of administering the drug is available?
   a. Topically
   b. Sublingually (under the tongue) or buccally (between the gums and cheek)
   c. Parenterally
   d. Nasally (by spray or NG tube)

10. Which antifungal drug is associated with hair loss?
    a. Flucytosine (Ancobon)
    b. Ketoconazole
    c. Griseofulvin
    d. Terbinafine (Lamisil)

7 Drugs for Viral and Retroviral Infections

FILL IN THE BLANK

Select the correct term from the list below.

- cART (combination antiretroviral therapy)
- virions
- retrovirus
- antivirals
- AIDS
- HIV
- viruses
- antiretrovirals

1. _____ drugs are used in treating the patient infected with HIV or for adults and children at risk for acquiring HIV and AIDS.

2. The drug therapy for HIV and AIDS that combines different types of antiretroviral drugs to use together daily is known as _____.

3. _____ is the later stage of HIV disease that causes a breakdown in the immune system, leaving the patient unable to fight infection.

4. Drugs that are capable of interfering with the ability of the virus to carry out its reproductive functions are called _____.

5. The specific retrovirus, known as _____, is responsible for the immune system problems associated with destruction of helper T cells (CD4 cells) when the infection results in disease and progresses to AIDS.

VIRUS OR RETROVIRUS

Indicate whether each of the statements below describes a virus (V) or a retrovirus (R).

6. _____ Infectious agent that reproduces only inside other living cells

7. _____ Causes damage and eventual death of an infected cell

8. _____ Transmit their own information into a cell's DNA

9. _____ Surrounded by a protein or fatty coating known as a capsid

10. _____ Uses the host cell's metabolic systems to make new viral particles

IDENTIFYING ANTIVIRAL DRUGS

Match the drug(s) used to treat each of the following viruses.

11. _____ Herpes (HSV)

12. _____ Influenza

13. _____ CMV

14. _____ RSV

15. _____ HPB

16. _____ HVC

A. Acyclovir
B. Adefovir
C. Famciclovir
D. Foscarnet
E. Ribavirin
F. Ledipasvis
G. Amantadine
H. Entecavir
I. Penciclovir

ANTIVIRAL SIDE EFFECTS & ADVERSE REACTIONS

Place an X next to each of the following items that identify a common (NOT adverse) side effect that you must look for when a patient is being treated with an antiviral drug.

17. _____ Vomiting

18. _____ Kidney damage

19. _____ Depression

20. _____ Diarrhea

21. _____ Headache

22. _____ Reddened skin (when using topicals)

List at least two adverse effects from common antiviral drugs that you need to monitor if your patient is being treated for one of the following viruses.

23. Flu _____

24. Herpes _____

25. CMV _____

26. RSV _____

27. HPB _____

28. HVC _____

TEACHING PATIENTS AND FAMILIES ABOUT ANTIVIRALS

Fill in the blank for each of the topics below that describe the type of information patients and their families need to be aware of when taking antiviral drugs.

29. If using _____ cream, warn them the skin may become red and excessive use can cause systemic side effects.

30. Be aware of true _____ allergies.

31. Expected side effects to _____ include vomiting, nausea, diarrhea, or headache.

32. When using topical drugs for treatment of HSV-1 (cold sores) or HSV-2 (genital herpes), use gloves and wash your _____ thoroughly so the infection does not spread.

33. There is no cure for _____. Antivirals can only treat _____ prophylactically or symptomatically.

32

34. Check yourself (or your family member) _____ for worsening symptoms that may indicate pneumonia or bacterial infection.

35. Antivirals can also be used for prevention or prophylaxis of the _____ in unvaccinated persons who have been exposed to the disease.

36. Follow the specific _____ instructions for the drug listed on the package.

ANTIRETROVIRAL DRUGS MATCHING

Match the drug names with one of the six categories of antiretroviral therapy drugs. You may use the categories more than once.

Drugs

37. _____ Fosamprenavir

38. _____ Enfuvirtide

39. _____ Delavirdine

40. _____ Dolutegravir

41. _____ Abacavir

42. _____ Maraviroc

43. _____ Atazanavir

44. _____ Dolutegravir

45. _____ Efavirenz

Categories

A. nucleoside reverse transcriptase inhibitors
B. non-nucleoside reverse transcriptase inhibitors
C. protease inhibitors
D. integrase inhibitors
E. fusion inhibitors
F. entry inhibitors

Match the drug category(ies) with one (or more) cautions that patients and their families need to know about when taking drugs from each category.

Drugs

46. _____ Do not chew or crush because this causes the drug to be absorbed too rapidly.

47. _____ To avoid birth defects, do not take if pregnant.

48. _____ Avoid St. John's wort.

49. _____ Avoid fatty and fried foods.

50. _____ Take at least 1 hour before or 2 hours after taking an antacid.

51. _____ Watch for injection site reactions.

52. _____ Can cause hypotension

53. _____ May cause peripheral neuropathy

54. _____ Report jaundice; can cause liver toxicity

55. _____ Report cough, fever, etc.; can cause pneumonia

Categories

A. nucleoside reverse transcriptase inhibitors
B. non-nucleoside reverse transcriptase inhibitors
C. protease inhibitors
D. integrase inhibitors
E. fusion inhibitors
F. entry inhibitors

Fill in the blank for each of the topics below that describe the type of information patients and their families need to be aware of when taking retroantiviral drugs.

56. Take the drugs exactly as ordered every day to ensure the drugs work properly and your disease does not become _____ to the drugs.

57. Take the drugs at the same _____ every day and use a cell phone reminder for time alerts. This way, drug levels remains steady and viral suppression is ideal.

58. Alert your healthcare provider to specific symptoms that may indicate _____ reactions immediately.

59. Safer _____ practice and standard precautions must be taken to prevent disease transmission.

60. Impaired immunity makes it more likely to contract diseases. Avoid eating raw _____ and fish, or fruits and vegetables that cannot be peeled or scrubbed.

61. If you are lactating, stop _____ your baby because there is a high risk of HIV transmission in breast milk.

62. Report any new OTC, herbs, _____, illegal drugs, and nutritional supplements to your prescriber because they could cause increased adverse reactions.

63. Avoid alcohol and recreational drugs because of the increased risk for _____ damage associated with these drugs.

64. Report signs of _____: numbness; tingling in feet or hands, which spreads to legs and arms; sharp, jabbing, throbbing, or burning pain in arms and legs; and decreased coordination and falling.

65. If you have symptoms of _____ (upper abdominal pain that may radiate to your back, pain that worsens after eating, increased nausea, and vomiting), notify your healthcare provider immediately so treatment can begin early.

CASE STUDIES

Walter Grantham is a 28-year-old man who has HIV. He has been taking antiretroviral drugs prescribed by his healthcare provider for almost a year. Walter arrives at the clinic presenting with upper abdominal pain with the pain radiating to his back. Walter says the pain worsens after he eats. He also states that his has had more nausea than usual and has vomited 3 times that day. Upon examining Walter, you find he has a temperature of 101 and has a resting pulse rate of 108.

1. What could be causing Walter's symptoms? (Choose the correct answer.)
   a. Gastroenteritis
   b. Pancreatitis
   c. Gallbladder stones
   d. Stomach ulcers

2. What should be your course of action? (Select all that apply.)
   a. Confirm with the healthcare provider that Walter's symptoms may indicate pancreatitis.
   b. Prescribe an antibiotic and ask Walter to return in 7 days if symptoms are not gone.
   c. Walter should immediately be taken to the hospital because pancreatitis is a medical emergency.
   d. Schedule an exploratory surgical consultation with a surgeon.
   e. Review his medications and ensure he is taking his drugs appropriately.
   f. Do a history to determine if he has been sexually active lately.

Doris Smith, a 68-year-old woman, walks into your clinic with what appears to be a case of influenza. She has fever and chills and her throat feels raw. She reports that yesterday she felt fine but woke up feeling ill and came to the clinic as soon as possible. The primary care provider wants to prescribe Zanamivir.

3. Why might the primary care provider choose Zanamivir?
   a. Because the patient is over 60 years of age.
   b. Because her throat feels raw.
   c. Because her symptoms were caught early.
   d. Because she had requested that drug.

4. When doing her history, what do you need to know specifically about Doris Smith before the drug can be prescribed? (Select all that apply.)
   a. Does she have an allergy to milk?
   b. Does she have an allergy to soy?
   c. What other drugs is she taking?
   d. Did she have the influenza vaccination this year?
   e. Does she have asthma?
   f. Has she had the pneumonia vaccine within the last 2 years?

PRACTICE QUIZ

1. Which of the following statements most accurately states the purpose of both antiviral and antiretroviral drugs?
   a. If started at the earliest onset of the infection, these drugs can cure the patient who has a virus or retrovirus.
   b. Because of the many side effects and adverse reactions, most healthcare providers are reluctant to prescribe these drugs.
   c. Patients who have been treated with antiviral or antiretroviral drugs once, cannot continue if a second outbreak occurs.
   d. Antiviral and antiretroviral drugs limit or slow the advance of the virus or retrovirus but do not cure the patient.

2. What does combination antiretroviral therapy, or cART, indicate for a patient?
   a. Several types of antiretroviral drugs are used together daily for patients infected by HIV.
   b. Different antiretroviral drugs are administered each day of the week, and then the routine is repeated on the following week.
   c. This method is used for individuals who are at high risk for HIV infection.
   d. Combination antiretroviral therapy, or cART, is utilized to prevent attachment of the HIV retrovirus to the outside of the CD4 cell.

3. Which of the following groups of individuals are at the lowest risk for developing HIV infection?
   a. Transgender women who have sex with men
   b. Women, who are White and have sex with other women
   c. Minority heterosexual women
   d. Intravenous drug users

4. Which category of antiretroviral drug is given early in the life cycle of an HIV infection?
   a. Protease inhibitors
   b. Fusion inhibitors
   c. Nucleoside reverse transcriptase inhibitors
   d. Entry inhibitors

5. Who is eligible to receive pre-exposure prophylaxis drug therapy?
   a. Persons who had sex with an individual who is in the early stages of HIV infection
   b. Healthcare personnel who work extensively with patients who are HIV positive
   c. Sex partners of persons who are HIV positive and using cART
   d. Men who regularly have sex with other men

6. One of the adverse reactions to antivirals and antiretroviral drug therapy is pancreatitis. Which is one of the signs or symptoms of pancreatitis?
   a. Upper abdominal pain or pain that radiates to your back
   b. Pain that lessens after eating
   c. Abnormally slow pulse and blood pressure
   d. Jaundiced skin

7. In the U.S. and Canada, what is one of the most common ways hepatitis B and hepatitis C are transmitted?
   a. Contaminated water
   b. Sexual activity
   c. Spoiled meat
   d. Respiratory infections

8. Although the cost is prohibitive for most individuals, what new drug may represent a cure for hepatitis C?
   a. Harvoni
   b. Virazole
   c. Hepsera
   d. Interferon

9. Which are the only two antivirals approved for treating or preventing influenza in children? (Select two.)
   a. Rapivab
   b. Relenza
   c. Amantadin
   d. Tamiflu

10. There are seven steps in the HIV life cycle. At which phase does HIV change the CD4 cell's DNA and the RNA messenger and cause the CD4 cell to start making long HIV protein chains?
    a. Replication
    b. Budding
    c. Integration
    d. Assembly

11. Why are the six categories of antiretroviral drugs referred to as inhibitors?
    a. They inhibit all other types of viruses and retroviruses from attacking the cells.
    b. They inhibit bodily functions from becoming overreactive to HIV.
    c. They suppress retroviral reproduction.
    d. They suppress white blood cell production.

12. How long must a patient continue combination antiretroviral drug therapy (cART)?
    a. Until the CD4 cell counts return to normal
    b. For approximately 35 years
    c. For the remainder of his or her life
    d. Until the budding phase of the life cycle is complete

35

13. During pregnancy, which category of antiretroviral drugs are commonly given to women who are HIV positive? (Select three.)
    a. Nucleoside reverse transcriptase inhibitors
    b. Non-nucleoside reverse transcriptase inhibitors
    c. Protease inhibitors
    d. Entry inhibitors
    e. Fusion inhibitors
    f. Integrase inhibitors

14. What is a sign indicating that the person who was HIV positive has developed full-blown AIDS?
    a. There is an increased number of CD4 cells in the body.
    b. The person develops allergic reactions to the antiretroviral drug therapy.
    c. There is a breakdown in the immune system in which the person is no longer able to fight any infection.
    d. The person is diagnosed with cancers such as pancreatic cancer.

15. Which virus is the common cause of chest colds, croup, and pneumonia in children?
    a. Influenza
    b. RSV
    c. CMV
    d. HPB

8 Drugs for Allergy and Respiratory Problems

IDENTIFYING TYPES OF DRUGS

Match the drug name with the category of drugs.

Drugs

1. _____ Albuterol
2. _____ Benzonatate
3. _____ Montelukast
4. _____ Guaifenesin
5. _____ Brompheniramine
6. _____ Fexofenadine
7. _____ Fluticasone
8. _____ Promethazine and codeine
9. _____ Ipratropium
10. _____ Zafirlukast
11. _____ Tiotropium
12. _____ Triamcinolone
13. _____ Arformoterol
14. _____ Levalbuterol
15. _____ Formoterol

Drug Categories

A. Antihistamines
B. Leukotriene inhibitors
C. Decongestants
D. Short acting beta$_2$ agonists
E. Long-acting beta$_2$ agonists
F. Cholinergic antagonists
G. Mucolytics
H. Antitussives

IDENTIFY THE CONDITION

For each of the following scenarios, identify what problem most likely describes what the client is experiencing.

16. Throughout the week, a newly admitted resident to a rehabilitation center experiences shortness of breath and has a dry, hacking cough. These incidents seem to occur every 3 to 4 days.

_____

17. A client who is recovering from bilateral knee replacement receives a bouquet of fragrant, blooming flowers. She immediately starts sneezing and her eyes begin to run.

_____

18. Your client seems to continually suffer from a chronic cough that produces clear, white, yellow, or green sticky mucus, wheezing, shortness of breath, and complains of chest tightness.

_____

FILL IN THE BLANK

19. _____ occur when the immune system develops a response to an environmental substance that it views as dangerous to the body.

20. _____ is a long-term condition of the airways that cause muscle constriction and inflammation of the airways and lungs. Symptoms are intermittent.

21. _____ is a progressive disease that obstructs air flow passages in the upper and lower airways. Constant inflammation produces large amounts of sticky mucus.

MULTIPLE CHOICE

For each of the drug types listed below, check all the statements that are applicable.

22. Antihistamines

_____ Could cause blindness

_____ Increase air flow through the bronchial tubes

_____ Reduce symptoms of sneezing, itching, and runny nose

_____ Could cause increased blood pressure

_____ Could cause slight nosebleed

_____ Drowsiness is an expected side effect

23. Leukotriene inhibitors

_____ Block histamines to prevent inflammation

_____ Decrease the thickness of respiratory secretions and aids in their removal

_____ Long-term use could lead to liver dysfunction

_____ Used to reduce symptoms of allergies and asthma

24. Decongestants

_____ Reduce the swelling of nasal passages

_____ Used to relieve or suppress coughing

_____ Overuse can cause insomnia

_____ Use daily for extended periods of time

25. Short-acting beta$_2$-adrenergic agonists (SABAs)

_____ Relaxe smooth muscles almost immediately

_____ Effects wear off quickly

_____ Common side effects include depression

_____ May cause tremors

26. Long-acting beta$_2$-adrenergic agonists

_____ May cause rising intraocular pressure

_____ Taken daily to prevent bronchospasms

_____ Orally inhaled and bind to beta$_2$-adrenergic receptors

_____ Dry mouth and bad taste are common side effects

27. Cholinergic antagonists

_____ Orally inhaled controller drugs

_____ Relax the muscles around the airways

_____ Allow more of the body's own adrenalin to activate beta$_2$ receptors

_____ May cause constipation

28. Mucolytics

_____ Shrink swollen nasal membranes

_____ May cause fungal infection in the nose or throat

_____ Prevent bronchoconstriction in asthma

_____ Decrease the thickness of respiratory secretions and aid in their removal

29. Antitussives

_____ Relieve or suppress coughing

_____ Can work by peripherally anesthetizing stretch receptors in the respiratory tract

_____ Capsules that are not swallowed whole can anesthetize the throat

_____ Prevents mast and white blood cells from releasing mediators of inflammation

FILL IN THE BLANKS

For the following teaching information for each drug type, fill in the blank with the appropriate word(s).

Antihistamines

30. Unless you must restrict your _____ intake because of another health problem, drink extra _____s to help prevent respiratory tract dryness.

31. Do not drink _____ while taking antihistamines because the CNS depressant effects of antihistamines may be increased.

32. Avoid _____ until you know how antihistamines affect you because they cause drowsiness in many clients.

33. If the drug causes _____ upset, take it with meals or milk to decrease this problem.

Leukotriene inhibitors

34. Report any increase in _____ attacks or allergic symptoms to your healthcare provider.

35. Consider not taking these drugs if you are _____ or breast feeding.

36. Because these drugs are used to prevent (rather than stop) _____ attacks or allergic responses, do not suddenly stop the drugs or decrease the dose.

Decongestants

37. Do not use sympathomimetic nasal _____ for more than 3 days because a rebound stuffiness and congestion are likely to occur.

38. If you have high blood pressure or heart problems, check with the pharmacist before using _____-_____-_____ cold preparations.

39. If you have _____ or cataracts, check with your healthcare provider before using corticosteroid nasal sprays.

40. Contact your healthcare provider if _____ patches develop in the nose or mouth while taking corticosteroid nasal sprays.

Beta-adrenergic agonists and anticholinergic antagonists

41. Contact your healthcare provider if bronchial _____, dizziness, chest pain, insomnia, or any changes in symptoms occur.

42. Drinking lots of fluid, especially water, makes the _____ thinner and helps the drug work better.

43. To prevent _____-induced bronchospasm, use your reliever bronchodilator inhaler 15 to 30 minutes before starting to _____.

44. After using your inhaler, rinse your mouth with _____ to decrease dry mouth and bad taste.

Mucolytic and antitussive drugs

45. Use a _____ and drink at least 2 quarts of water daily while taking a mucolytic unless there is a medical reason for fluid restriction. These actions will help get the mucus out.

46. Notify your healthcare provider if the cough is present with a high _____, rash, or persistent headaches, or if the cough returns once it has been under control.

47. Take the drug with at least one full glass of _____.

48. Do not take opioid antitussives with _____ or any other drugs that slow the central nervous system because the side effects will be intensified.

MATCHING

Indicate whether each of the steps below is referring to use of: a. metered dose inhaler, b. dry powder inhaler

49. _____ Insert the mouthpiece of the inhaler into the nonmouthpiece end of the spacer

50. _____ Turn the device to the next dose of drug.

51. _____ Fully exhale and then place the mouthpiece into your mouth, over your tongue.

52. _____ Never exhale (breathe out) into your inhaler.

53. _____ Never shake your inhaler.

54. _____ Breathe in slowly and deeply.

55. _____ Never wash or place the inhaler in water.

56. _____ Remove the mouthpiece from your mouth; keeping your lips closed, hold your breath for at least 10 seconds and then breathe out slowly.

57. _____ Place your lips over the mouthpiece and breathe in forcefully (there is no propellant in the inhaler; only your breath pulls the drug in).

58. _____ Wait at least 1 minute between puffs

59. _____ At least once a day, clean the case and cap of the inhaler.

60. _____ Exhale fully away from the inhaler.

CASE STUDIES

Faith Delacroix is a 40-year-old woman who came to the clinic stating she has been having difficulty breathing with a dry, nonproductive cough. She states she has been wheezing and short of breath even while talking. She was diagnosed with asthma several years ago but is presently not being treated. After discussing her asthma with the healthcare provider, you decide Faith should be assessed to determine if she needs a bronchodilator.

1. What would be included when assessing whether a patient with asthma needs a bronchodilator? (Select all that apply.)
   1. Is the client pregnant?
   2. Does the client have a history of liver disease?
   3. Take a baseline set of vital signs
   4. Is client breastfeeding?
   5. Obtain a stool sample
   6. Check for any history of hyperthyroidism, heart disease, hypertension, diabetes, glaucoma, seizures, or psychoneurotic disease.
   7. MRI of the lungs
   8. History of any allergies
   9. List of other drugs the client takes in case they would interact with bronchodilators

2. Choose the patient and family teaching points you would be responsible for providing if Faith is prescribed a bronchodilator for her asthma. (Select all that apply.)
   1. Take the drug as directed by the healthcare provider.
   2. The bronchodilator will make sputum more liquid and easier to spit out but will not help the cough.
   3. Overuse of these drugs may result in severe side effects.
   4. Contact your healthcare provider if the drug is not helping your breathing problems.
   5. Use a humidifier.
   6. Contact your healthcare provider if bronchial irritation, dizziness, chest pain, insomnia, or any change in symptoms occur.
   7. Drinking lots of fluid, especially water, makes the mucus thinner and helps the drug work better.
   8. Notify your healthcare provider if the cough is present with a high fever, rash, or persistent headaches, or if the cough returns once it has been under control.
   9. Change positions slowly when moving from a lying or sitting position.
   10. Do not take any OTC drugs without first checking with your healthcare provider.
   11. To prevent exercise-induced bronchospasm, use your reliever bronchodilator inhaler 15 to 30 minutes before starting to exercise.

1. Which of the following are considered harmless substances that can cause allergic reactions to people who are overly sensitive to them?
   a. Sand and dirt
   b. Dust mites
   c. Concrete parking lots
   d. Iron fences

2. Allergic reactions usually occur at the point of contact with the allergen. If the skin reacts to an allergen and becomes red and/or swollen, what is one common method of drug administration that can be used to lessen the reaction?
   a. Nasal spray
   b. Lung inhalation
   c. Topical cream
   d. Suppository

3. There are two types of histamines, H1 and H2. Antihistamines that block H1 receptors limit bronchoconstriction. What do antihistamines block when focused on H2 receptors?
   a. Skin irritation
   b. Lymph nodes
   c. Stomach acid production
   d. Nasal passage swelling

4. How can an individual procure first-generation antihistamines?
   a. With a prescription from an allergy specialist
   b. Can be purchased over the counter
   c. Are available over the Internet from Canada or India
   d. These drugs are no longer produced.

5. When assessing clients prior to administering antihistamines, what specific information should you obtain?
   a. Determine whether the client is actually allergic to the substance
   b. Examine the client's ears and throats to determine how badly affected they are from the allergic reaction
   c. Ask whether the client has objections due to religious reasons for taking any kind of medication
   d. Ask whether the client suffers from thyroid disease or migraine headaches

6. When should leukotriene inhibitors not be administered?
   a. If the client is having an acute asthma attack
   b. When the client is having an acute asthma attack
   c. Only to a client who has never had asthma
   d. Only to adults with asthma who weigh over 100 pounds

7. How do cromones reduce symptoms of clients with allergies or asthma?
   a. Block leukotriene response
   b. Activate mast cells that control the immune system
   c. Prevent mast cells from opening
   d. Prevent allergic responses to dander

8. What is the function of sympathomimetic drugs?
   a. Mimic stimulation of sympathetic nervous system and shrink blood vessels so the nose can drain more efficiently
   b. Block the body's adrenalin to reduce inflammation in the nasal passages
   c. Slow the production of histamine and leukotriene
   d. Reduce discomfort of skin allergies

9. Which of the following conditions does NOT prohibit use of oral sympathomimetic drugs?
   a. High blood pressure
   b. HIV
   c. Sinus infection
   d. Nasal inflammation

10. Why do clients with asthma usually require more than one type of drug to manage the symptoms?
    a. Many drugs become ineffective after long-term usage.
    b. Inflammation narrows airways from the inside and bronchoconstriction narrows airways from the outside.
    c. Asthma attacks are initiated by allergens and multiple drugs are necessary to focus on specific allergic reactions.
    d. To address the multiple symptoms of asthma (shortness of breath, wheezing, cough, etc.)

11. What is one of the usual causes of chronic obstructive pulmonary disease (COPD)?
    a. Allergies to dust mites
    b. Pneumonia
    c. Cigarette smoking
    d. Repeated bouts of bronchitis

12. Drug therapy for both asthma and COPD includes two types of agents. One agent is an antiinflammatory. What is the other type of agent required for treatment?
    a. Bronchodilator
    b. Sympathomimetic
    c. Corticosteroid
    d. Mast cell stabilizer

13. How do mucolytic drugs decrease the thickness of respiratory secretions?
   a. Enabling clients to cough up large quantities of thick mucus
   b. Increasing the amount of fluid in the respiratory tract
   c. Increasing the size of nasal passages to allow for more productive cough
   d. Enabling clients to drain sinuses more efficiently

14. According to the FDA, mucolytic drugs should not be given to which of the following clients?
   a. Immunocompromised clients
   b. Elderly clients
   c. Young children
   d. Pregnant or breastfeeding women

15. How do nonopioid antitussives reduce the cough reflex?
   a. Anesthetizing stretch receptors in respiratory passages, lungs, and pleura
   b. Acting directly on the cough center in the medulla of the brain
   c. Thinning the secretions to promote ciliary action
   d. Relaxing the muscles around the airway

16. SABAs and corticosteroid inhalers are often prescribed together to prevent bronchospasms. When using together, what is important to remember?
   a. SABAs are slow acting so do not help during an acute attack.
   b. SABAs can be combined with an inhaled corticosteroid in one inhaler.
   c. Always use the SABA inhaler first to open the airway and allow the corticosteroid to reach the respiratory tract.
   d. Some people feel "nervous" and may have tremors with these drugs.

9 Drugs Affecting the Renal/Urinary and Cardiovascular Systems

IDENTIFYING DRUGS BY USE

Match the drug name with its use.

Drugs

1. _____ hydrochlorothiazide

2. _____ quinidine

3. _____ simvastatin

4. _____ nitroglycerin

5. _____ trospium chloride

6. _____ tamsulosin

7. _____ quinapril

Drug Use

A. Diuretic
B. Benign prostatic hyperplasia
C. Overactive bladder
D. HMG-CoA reductase inhibitor (statin)
E. Antihypertensive
F. Antianginal
G. Antidysrhythmic

DRUG CATEGORIES

Match the description with each of the drug categories.

Description

8. _____ Slows the conduction of impulses through the heart

9. _____ Relaxes smooth muscle tissue in the prostate gland, the neck of the bladder, and the urethra by binding to the alpha-1 adrenergic receptors, placing less pressure on the urethra and improving urine flow

10. _____ Lowers blood LDL levels by slowing liver production of cholesterol

11. _____ Lowers blood pressure by increasing urine output and preventing water, sodium, potassium, and chloride from being reabsorbed back into the blood

12. _____ Decreases blood pressure by relaxing vascular smooth muscle in the coronary and systemic arteries, leading to decreased peripheral resistance

13. _____ Increases oxygen to the heart enabling it to pump more easily

14. _____ Inhibits involuntary nerve-induced contractions of the detrusor muscle, relaxing the bladder and holding more urine

Drug Categories

A. Thiazides
B. Selective alpha-1 blockers
C. Urinary antispasmodics
D. HMG-CoA reductase inhibitors (statins)
E. Calcium channel blockers
F. Nitrates
G. Sodium channel blockers

IDENTIFYING SIDE EFFECTS/ADVERSE EFFECTS

15. Which of the following are side effects and/or adverse effects of diuretic drugs? Check all that apply.
    a. _____ Urinary urgency and urinary frequency
    b. _____ Flare-ups of gout
    c. _____ Low magnesium
    d. _____ Dehydration

16. Which of the following are side-effects and/or adverse effects of HMG-CoA reductase inhibitors (statins)? Check all that apply.
    a. _____ Acid reflux
    b. _____ Sore throat
    c. _____ Jaundice
    d. _____ Muscle breakdown

17. Which of the following are side-effects and/or adverse effects of nonstatin antihyperlipidemic drugs? Check all that apply.
   a. _____ Gemfibrozil and fenofibrate can cause kidney failure and *cholelithiasis* (gallstones).
   b. _____ Bile acid sequestrants increase absorption of fat-soluble vitamins (A, D, E, and K),
   c. _____ Niacin use can cause *flushing* (red color in the face and neck).
   d. _____ Bile acid sequestrants can cause blood-clotting.

18. Which of the following are side-effects and/or adverse effects of antihypertensive drugs? Check all that apply.
   a. _____ Calcium channel blockers also work as diuretics.
   b. _____ Beta blockers can cause bronchoconstriction, which is a problem for patients with asthma.
   c. _____ Most antihypertensive drugs can cause dizziness when the patient changes positions.
   d. _____ Patients may experience a dramatic drop in blood pressure.

19. Which of the following are side-effects and/or adverse effects of nitrates? Check all that apply.
   a. _____ Throbbing headaches caused by rapid blood vessel dilation in the head can occur.
   b. _____ Severe postural hypertension when a person suddenly stands up
   c. _____ Reflex tachycardia (rapid heartbeat) or paradoxical bradycardia
   d. _____ Vitamin B deficiency

20. Which of the following are side-effects and/or adverse effects of inotropic drugs? Check all that apply.
   a. _____ These drugs can produce toxins within the body.
   b. _____ Symptoms of toxins include allergic reactions to nuts and dairy.
   c. _____ Early signs of toxins in infants and elderly include an unusually rapid heartbeat.
   d. _____ Children often experience hyperactivity and euphoria.

DESCRIBE PATIENT AND FAMILY TEACHING

For each of the following drug types, following the example provided, list at least three items you should teach patients and families regarding drug use.

21. Diuretics
   ■ Take the drug exactly as prescribed. Do not skip or double doses.
   Your responses

22. HMG-CoA reductase inhibitors (statins)
   ■ Lifestyle changes like exercise, a low cholesterol diet, and good weight management are just as important while you are taking the statins to help prevent cardiovascular disease.
   Your responses

23. Niacin or nicotinic acid
   ■ Take the drug at the time prescribed because timing is important for cholesterol-lowering drugs.
   Your responses

24. Antihypertensive drugs
   - Take this drug exactly as ordered. If a dose is missed, it should be taken as soon as it is remembered; if it is close to the next scheduled dose, skip the missed dose and return to the regular dosing schedule.
   Your responses

25. Antianginals
   - Keep the nitroglycerin (NTG) tablets in a dark glass container to prevent breakdown of the drug.
   Your responses

26. Antidysrhythmics
   - Take this drug exactly as ordered and do not skip doses or double the dose.
   Your responses

27. Inotropic Drugs
   - Let your healthcare provider know if you have any loss of appetite, nausea, vomiting, diarrhea, or any vision changes that can be an indication of digoxin toxicity.
   Your responses

CASE STUDIES

Shawn Murphy is a 78-year-old man who suffers with coronary heart disease. He had one heart attack 3 years ago. He has not changed his diet nor does he get enough exercise. He has been experiencing some angina, especially when he exerts himself physically. The healthcare provider prescribes sublingual nitroglycerin (NTG) for acute attacks and transdermal nitroglycerin patches to reduce the frequency and severity of the angina.

1. What should you teach Mr. Murphy to do in the case of an acute angina attack? (Select all that apply.)
   1. Place the NTG tablet under his tongue as soon as the pain starts
   2. Do not chew or swallow the tablet
   3. Only touch NTG tablets when wearing gloves to avoid it being absorbed into the bloodstream
   4. Tell Mr. Murphy to lie down while the tablet dissolves
   5. Instruct Mr. Murphy to call 911 or go to the emergency room if pain has not subsided in 5 minutes
   6. Blood pressure checks are essential before taking the second NTG tablet
   7. Do not drive
   8. Common side effects are nausea, vomiting, and blurred vision
   9. Mr. Murphy can take a second pill while waiting for emergency services
   10. If pain has not subsided in another 5 minutes. Mr. Murphy may take a third pill
   11. Do not take more than three NTG tablets
   12. Drinking coffee with the tablet is recommended

45

2. What type of monitoring and evaluation will Mr. Murphy need while taking NTG, both sublingual and transdermal? (Choose all that apply.)
    1. Blood pressure checks every five minutes after taking a NTG tablet for acute angina
    2. Schedule blood lipid levels, ordered by the prescriber, every 4–12 weeks
    3. Have Mr. Murphy report frequency and severity of headaches
    4. Tell Mr. Murphy to never drink grapefruit juice with nitrates
    5. Plan with Mr. Murphy when he will have an "off" time for the transdermal patches
    6. Do not give NTG if Mr. Murphy's blood pressure is less than 90/60 mm Hg
    7. Check Mr. Murphy for jaundice

Susan Rice is a 70-year-old woman with congestive heart failure. Among other medications, she taking 2 mg of Bumex on a daily basis. She comes to the clinic for her regular check-up. She reports symptoms of dry mouth, muscle cramps, and weakness.

3. Based of Mrs. Rice's symptoms and that she is taking Bumex, what do you suspect may be her problem?
    1. Low potassium
    2. Low blood sugar
    3. High potassium
    4. High blood sugar

4. The healthcare provider orders a blood test. What are you specifically looking for on her test that will support the suspected problem?
    1. Potassium level less than 3.5 mEq/L
    2. Blood sugar level less than 65 mg/dL
    3. Potassium level greater than 6 mEq/L
    4. Blood sugar level greater than 140 mg/dL

PRACTICE QUIZ

1. How do the renal/urinary systems and the cardiovascular system work together to maintain adequate circulation in the body?
    a. The two systems ensure the bowels work efficiently.
    b. The two systems help maintain fluid balance.
    c. The two systems regulate heartbeat.
    d. The two systems regulate what comes into the kidneys.

2. Your elderly patient is taking a diuretic. What side effects do you need to watch for, other than dehydration?
    a. Signs of low potassium
    b. Unusually dry skin
    c. Magnesium deficiency
    d. Change in urine color

3. What symptoms are controlled by phenazopyridine?
    a. Cures urinary tract infection
    b. Treats infections causing irritation to the bladder
    c. Manages color of the urine
    d. Controls burning and pain of the urinary tract

4. Which of the following conditions can cause ischemia?
    a. Dehydration due to overuse of diuretics
    b. Decreased blood flow through the coronary arteries
    c. Decreased kidney output
    d. Increased blood flow through the coronary arteries

5. How is heart failure usually managed in order to reduce associated symptoms?
    a. Depending on other health conditions, the patient is put on list for transplant
    b. Patients increase heart function through diet and exercise
    c. Patients are administered a variety of cardiovascular drugs
    d. Patients are administered antibiotics to ensure optimum systemic health

6. Why should grapefruit juice not be used when a patient is administered statins?
    a. Increases liver toxicity
    b. Increases concentrations in blood, promoting toxic side effects
    c. Decreases the effectiveness of statins, resulting in poor performance
    d. Causes anaphylactic shock in some patients

7. How does ezetimibe lower cholesterol?
    a. Limits the absorption of cholesterol from food or other sources
    b. Destroys cholesterol cells attached to the intestinal wall
    c. Blocks cholesterol from entering the cardiac system
    d. Limits the ability of cholesterol cells to reproduce within the body

8. The Joint National Committee on the Prevention, Detection, Evaluation, and Treatment of High Blood Pressure recommends best practices for hypertension management. Before beginning drug therapy, what does the Commission recommend as the first attempt in reducing hypertension?
    a. Stress reduction
    b. Vitamin supplements
    c. Surgical intervention
    d. Lifestyle modification

9. Before teaching a patient about possible changes they can make to reduce their high blood pressure, you need to assess modifiable and nonmodifiable risk factors. Which of the following is a non-modifiable risk factor?
   a. Smoking
   b. Levels of physical activity
   c. Race
   d. Diet

10. What is the usual cause of a myocardial infarction?
    a. Comorbidities such as renal failure
    b. Rapid heartbeat on a daily basis
    c. Reduction of blood flow to the heart muscle
    d. Niacin deficiency

11. You should not administer nitroglycerin if your patient's blood pressure goes below which of the following readings?
    a. 90/60
    b. 110/60
    c. 120/65
    d. 100/70

12. Which term is used to describe irregular heartbeat rhythm?
    a. Arrhythmia
    b. Dysrhythmia
    c. Angithythmia
    d. Cardiothythmia

13. When assessing a patient before giving digoxin, which must you check for?
    a. Ensure the patient is getting sufficient oxygen to the blood stream
    b. Ensure the patient's heart rate is 59 or below
    c. Ensure the patient's heart rate is 60 or above
    d. Ensure that patient's magnesium level is normal

14. How can you monitor a nursing home patient who is taking diuretics to ensure he doesn't become dehydrated?
    a. Weigh the patient on a daily basis
    b. Test the skin for flexibility
    c. Ensure the patient drinks 64 ounces of water per day
    d. Record each time the patient urinates and monitor the amount

15. Should statins be administered in the evening or in the morning?
    a. All statins should be administered in the morning.
    b. It does not matter what time of day statins are administered as long as they are taken consistently.
    c. It varies by the type of drug prescribed.
    d. It is preferable to administer statins at bedtime.

10 Drugs for Central Nervous System Problems

DRUGS FOR PARKINSON'S DISEASE

FILL IN THE BLANKS

1. Parkinson's disease is a disorder of the central nervous system and indicates a lack of _____.

2. Without dopamine, movements become hard to control and some muscles are _____.

3. Arms and legs "catch" at certain points in a "stop-and-go" fashion known as _____ rigidity.

4. Other symptoms include "masklike" facial features, risk for falls, tremors, and difficulty chewing, swallowing, and _____.

5. Frequent complications include _____, hallucinations, and anxiety.

MATCHING

Match the items on the left, which include related drug names, descriptions, and administration details, with the Parkinson's disease drug types on the right. You will use each drug type more than once.

Drug Information

6. _____ Entacapone

7. _____ Safinamide

8. _____ Increase dopamine levels of the brain

9. _____ Patients should avoid foods/beverages containing large amounts of tyramine

10. _____ Carbidopa/levodopa tablets

11. _____ High-protein foods decrease absorption

12. _____ Allow existing dopamine to remain active in the brain longer

13. _____ Pramipexole

14. _____ Help dopamine and dopamine agonist drugs to remain active in the body longer

15. _____ Administer 30–60 minutes before meals

16. _____ May turn urine to orange brown color

17. _____ Rasagiline

18. _____ Administer these drugs at the same time every day

19. _____ Tolcapone

20. _____ Sinemet

Drug Types

A. Dopamine agonists
B. Catechol-O-methyltransferase (COMT) inhibitors
C. Selective monoamine oxidase B (MAO-B) inhibitors

TRUE OR FALSE

Indicate whether each of the following statements regarding side effects/adverse reactions to drugs that treat the symptoms Parkinson's disease are true (T) or false (F)

21. _____ One of the most common side effects of carbidopa/levodopa and all dopamine agonists is the eruption of cold sores around the mouth.

22. _____ The most common adverse reaction to Rytary is dyskinesia.

23. _____ If a patient is taking dopamine agonists and suffers from delirium, psychosis, or hallucinations, this is related to the disease process, not the drug.

24. _____ As carbidopa/levodopa dosages decrease when COMT inhibitors and MAO-B inhibitors are added to the drug regime, the patient could experience neuroleptic malignant syndrome.

25. _____ The effectiveness of dopamine agonists is reduced when taken with a steak dinner.

SHORT ANSWER

26. When is the best time to administer dopamine agonists in conjunction with meals or snacks?

27. If the patient is taking levodopa, which vitamin is contraindicated because it accelerates the inactivation of the drug?

28. Approximately how soon will you begin to see clinical improvements in a patient who begins taking drugs to treat the symptoms of Parkinson's disease?

29. When taking MAO-B inhibitors, what are some of the symptoms which if suddenly worsen indicate you should contact the healthcare provider immediately?

30. What instructions should you give to your patients to help them avoid falling due to low blood pressure, which can result from drugs used to treat the symptoms of Parkinson's disease?

DRUGS FOR ALZHEIMER'S DISEASE

FILL IN THE BLANK

1. Alzheimer's disease is one of many forms of _____, which is the progressive loss of brain function.

2. Alzheimer's disease causes changes to multiple aspects of the brain; over time, these changes _____ the size of the brain and all aspects of brain function.

3. Drugs, including cholinesterase inhibitors and NMDA blockers, provide _____ improvement in symptoms.

4. Symptoms of Alzheimer's disease begin with memory issues which get progressively worse and eventually include confusion and changes in mood, judgment, and _____.

5. When evaluating a patient for Alzheimer's disease, it is important to know the risk factors, which include age greater than 65, family history, and having the APOE-e4 _____.

MATCHING

Match the items on the left, which include related drug names, descriptions, and administration details, with the Alzheimer's disease drug types on the right. You will use each drug type more than once.

Drug Information

6. _____ Bind to acetylcholinesterase enzyme and slows its breakdown of acetylcholine

7. _____ Galantamine

8. _____ Memantine

9. _____ Donepezil

10. _____ Adverse effects include somnolence

11. _____ Monitor patients taking these drugs for worsening asthma conditions and GI bleeds

12. _____ Reduce neuronal damage by protecting neurons from calcium

Drug Types

A. Cholinesterase inhibitors
B. NMDA (N-methyl-D-aspartate) blockers

TRUE OR FALSE

Indicate whether each of the following statements regarding drugs that treat the symptoms of Alzheimer's disease are true (T) or false (F).

13. _____ If Alzheimer's disease is diagnosed at an early stage, a combination of cholinesterase inhibitors and NMDA blockers can alleviate the disease entirely.

14. _____ Aricept should be taken at bedtime.

15. _____ Patients taking cholinesterase inhibitors should urinate every 2 hours to prevent incontinence.

16. _____ NMDA blockers that come in extended release capsules must be taken whole.

17. _____ If using a liquid form of NMDA blockers, it can be mixed with other liquids to improve taste.

18. _____ If a patient is taking NMDA blockers, it is important to monitor the patient's blood pressure.

SHORT ANSWER

19. What is one adverse effect applicable to both cholinesterase inhibitors and NMDA blockers?

20. To evaluate a patient for symptom improvement before he starts a cholinesterase inhibitor, how should you assess him?

21. Why should you assess a patient for swallowing difficulties?

22. Why should patients with risk for renal impairment be cautioned prior to taking memantine?

DRUGS FOR EPILEPSY

FILL IN THE BLANK

1. Epilepsy is a type of chronic _____ disorder in which brain neurons become hyperexcitable and trigger unneeded electrical signals.

2. Seizures are the body's response to those inappropriate _____ signals.

3. A _____ is the sudden contraction of many muscle groups without the person's conscious control.

4. Based on symptoms, length, and degree of consciousness, seizures are classified first as _____ or generalized.

TRUE OR FALSE

Indicate whether each of the following statements regarding drugs that treat the symptoms of epilepsy are true (T) or false (F).

5. _____ Phenytoin can be used safely with patients who are pregnant.

6. _____ Carbamazepine use increases a patient's risk of sunburn.

7. _____ Phenobarbital can cause depression of the central nervous system.

8. _____ Valproic acid is not recommended for patients who are diagnosed with COPD due to the possibility of depression of the respiratory system.

9. _____ Amnesia is a potential adverse reaction to lamotrigine.

10. _____ Lacosamide has been known to cause euphoria in patients and is therefore sometimes given as an antidepressant.

11. _____ Topiramine use is associated with memory loss.

CROSSWORD PUZZLE

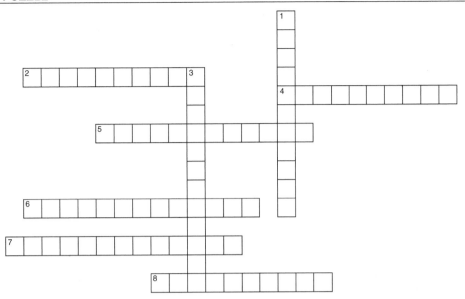

ACROSS

2. Appears to stabilize neuron membranes and prevent repetitive excitation and firing
4. Appears to reduce seizures by preventing spread of excitation in brain GABA
5. Increases the activity of the inhibitory neurotransmitter GABA
6. Enhances the action of the inhibitory neurotransmitter
7. Limits spread of neuron excitation by altering the sodium channels of nerve membranes
8. Prevents spread of neuron excitation binding to sodium channels on nerve membranes

DOWN

1. Unknown action thought to reduce seizures by blocking sodium
3. Reduces seizures by altering calcium channels on the neuron membrane

MATCHING

Match the patient teaching descriptions on the left with the epilepsy drug on the right. You may use each drug type more than once.

Teaching Descriptions

12. _____ Warn patient to note symptoms of metabolic acidosis such as slow heart rate and warm, flushed skin

13. _____ Can cause bradycardia, so take pulse daily and report changes and irregularities

14. _____ Check daily for rashes

15. _____ Ask provider if folic acid supplements are needed

16. _____ Increases risk of falls

17. _____ Can cause tachycardia, so take pulse daily and report changes and irregularities

18. _____ Do not increase dosage to improve mood-enhancing properties

19. _____ Take with meals to avoid GI distress

20. _____ Use good oral hygiene to prevent gum disease

21. _____ Note changes in respiratory functions

22. _____ Parents should observe children for signs of yellowing skin

23. _____ Report headaches and muscle weakness, which could be signs of low sodium

24. _____ Warn patient to note symptoms of encephalopathys such as lethargy or vomiting

25. _____ May be used when pregnant

Drugs

A. Phenytoins
B. Carbamazepine
C. Ethosuximide
D. Phenobarbital
E. Valproic acid
F. Oxcarbazepine
G. Lamotrigine
H. Lacosamide
I. Topiramine

DRUGS FOR MULTIPLE SCLEROSIS

FILL IN THE BLANK

1. Multiple sclerosis (MS) is an autoimmune disease affecting the _____ in the brain and spinal cord.

2. Symptoms of multiple sclerosis occur when the nerve transmission is _____.

3. Multiple sclerosis is more common in _____ than _____.

4. Multiple sclerosis cannot be cured, but drug therapy can slow _____.

5. In the past, there were no specific drugs for treatment of MS; therefore, patient drug therapy consisted of anti-inflammatories, such as _____.

6. Biological response modifiers modify the MS patient's response to abnormal _____ for immunity and inflammation.

7. Monoclonal antibodies for MS attack and either inactivate or destroy _____ that damage the myelin.

8. Neurologic drugs for MS either protect nerves and myelin from destruction or improve impulse _____ of demyelinated nerves.

MATCHING

Match the drug for relapsing-remitting multiple sclerosis on the left with the drug types on the right. You may use each drug type more than once.

Drug Names

9. _____ Dimethyl fumarate

10. _____ Beta-interferon

11. _____ Ocrelizumab

12. _____ Dalfampridine

13. _____ Alemtuzumab

14. _____ Fingolimod

Drug Types

A. Biological response modifiers
B. Monoclonal antibodies
C. Neurologic drugs

SYMPTOMS

Select which of the symptoms are associated with each of the multiple sclerosis drug types.

15. Biological response modifiers
   - ☐ Earache
   - ☐ Peripheral neuropathy
   - ☐ Increased UTIs
   - ☐ Slow heart rate
   - ☐ Thinning scalp hair

16. Monoclonal antibodies
   - ☐ Increased risk for infection
   - ☐ Higher risk for pneumonia
   - ☐ Foot pain
   - ☐ Hypertension
   - ☐ Edema

17. Neurologic drugs
   - ☐ Headache, dizziness, muscle weakness
   - ☐ GI problems, heartburn, constipation
   - ☐ Confusion, seizure activity
   - ☐ Nausea, diarrhea, abdominal pain
   - ☐ Flushing, itching, rashes

DRUGS FOR AMYOTROPHIC LATERAL SCLEROSIS (ALS)

FILL IN THE BLANKS

1. ALS is a progressive, fatal _____ disease that affects the motor nerves of the brain and spinal cord.

2. The disease ALS can strike anyone at any time; however, it usually affects persons between the ages of _____ and _____.

3. Loss of _____ is usually the first symptom of the disease.

4. It is known that ALS patients have excess _____ in both their brain and spinal cord.

5. Riluzole, a _____, reduces the actions of glutamate by either inhibiting or blocking the action and/or release of glutamate.

SHORT ANSWER

6. What are the most frequently expected side effects of riluzole?

7. Name two drugs that should be used with caution when administering riluzole.

MATCHING

Match the following statements with the correct category of Nursing Implications and Patient Teaching

8. _____ Riluzole should be administered at least 1 hour before or 2 hours after a meal.

9. _____ Liver function enzymes should be monitored before and during the course of therapy every month for first 3 months, every 3 months for remainder of the first year, and periodically as needed after that.

10. _____ Driving or engaging in potentially hazardous activities until the response to the drug is known is dangerous and should not be undertaken.

11. _____ If a febrile illness develops, the WBC count should be monitored because neutropenia can occur with this drug.

12. _____ Differentiating between the adverse side effects and the actions of riluzole is difficult because the manifestations of ALS (weakness and lack of energy) are often associated with side effects.

13. _____ Do not drink alcohol while taking this drug, as potential adverse effects exist.

14. _____ Several cases of interstitial lung disease have been reported with riluzole, so check with the healthcare provider if the patient has pulmonary disease.

15. _____ Driving or engaging in potentially hazardous activities until the response to the drug is known is dangerous and should not be undertaken.

16. _____ Withhold the drug and notify the healthcare provider if liver enzymes are elevated.

17. _____ Riluzole should be administered at least 1 hour before or 2 hours after a meal.

18. _____ If a febrile illness develops, the WBC count should be monitored because neutropenia can occur with this drug.

A. Assessment
B. Planning and Implementation
C. Evaluation
D. Patient and Family Teaching

DRUGS FOR MYASTHENIA GRAVIS (MG)

FILL IN THE BLANKS

1. Myasthenia gravis is an _____ disease that attacks the neuromuscular junction, which is the connection between the nerve and muscle.

2. The disease is more prevalent in women younger than _____ years old and men older than _____ years old.

3. Often, eye _____ and double vision are the first signs of disease, as the eye muscles are among the first to be affected.

4. Other symptoms include arm and leg weakness, _____, and difficulty with chewing, swallowing, and breathing.

5. The muscles become weaker as they are _____; consequently muscle weakness and fatigue are worse in the afternoon and evening.

SHORT ANSWER

6. What is the function of acetylcholine?

7. Which enzymes break down acetylcholine in the brain, causing weak muscles and fatigue?

8. Acetylcholine is the neurotransmitter that is released by what?

9. Patients test positive for myasthenia gravis if their muscles get stronger after being injected with what drug?

10. What drug is used for long-term maintenance of the disease?

EXPECTED SIDE EFFECTS/ADVERSE REACTIONS AND INTERACTIONS

11. Select all that apply.
    - ☐ Nausea
    - ☐ Hepatoxicity
    - ☐ Bradycardia and other dysrhythmias
    - ☐ Hypotension
    - ☐ Inflammation
    - ☐ Diarrhea
    - ☐ Vomiting
    - ☐ Respiratory distress and/or arrest
    - ☐ Lethargy and confusion
    - ☐ Increased bronchial secretions
    - ☐ Tricyclic antidepressants may antagonize some of the effects of drugs that mimic or enhance the parasympathetic nervous system
    - ☐ Cardiac arrest
    - ☐ High blood ammonia levels
    - ☐ Stomach cramps
    - ☐ Electrolyte imbalances
    - ☐ Difficulty swallowing and increased saliva

MATCHING

Match the following statements with the correct category of Nursing implications and patient teaching.

12. _____ The duration of the drug action can vary with physical and emotional stress, and disease severity

13. _____ Space doses by at least 6 hours

14. _____ Monitor vital signs frequently, especially respiratory rate

15. _____ Report onset of rash to the healthcare provider

16. _____ Pyridostigmine should be used with caution in patients with bronchial asthma, chronic obstructive pulmonary disease (COPD), bradycardia, or cardiac arrhythmias

17. _____ Extended-release products should be swallowed whole and not crushed or chewed

18. _____ Patients being treated for hypertension or glaucoma with beta-adrenergic receptor blockers may be at risk for unopposed cholinergic activity

19. _____ Evaluate and report muscular weakness, cramps, or muscular fasciculations

20. _____ Sustained-release tablets can become spotted in appearance, but this does not affect the potency of the drug

A. Assessment
B. Planning and implementation
C. Evaluation
D. Patient and family teaching

CASE STUDIES

Sarah Lewis is a 48-year-old woman who has breast cancer and has been undergoing chemotherapy. During chemotherapy, she developed a blood clot that was treated with blood thinners. Months later, she suffered a brain bleed. A week later, she began to blank out for several minutes, followed by disorientation and confusion. This happened several times during the day and Sarah did not remember these episodes. A neurologist diagnosed her with absence seizures and prescribed lamotrigine.

1. What are some of the teaching points you need to tell the patient and family about using lamotrigine? (Check all that apply.)
   1. Check yourself every day for skin rashes.
   2. Keep all appointments for laboratory testing because the drug can cause electrolyte problems and decrease blood counts.
   3. If you are taking the extended-release form of the drug, swallow it whole and do not crush, open, or chew it.
   4. If your mouth becomes uncomfortably dry, chewing gum, sucking hard candy, and drinking more water may help the problem.
   5. Change positions slowly, especially when moving from a lying or sitting position to a standing position
   6. Do not drive or operate dangerous equipment if your vision is blurred or if you have double vision.

2. What are the drugs that may interact with lamotrigine? (Check all that apply.)
   1. cardiac drugs
   2. aspirin and acetaminophen
   3. drugs for psychiatric problems
   4. drugs for HIV
   5. oral contraceptives
   6. antifungal drugs
   7. drugs for tuberculosis
   8. proton pump inhibitors
   9. drugs for diabetes

Margaret Graham is a 74-year-old woman recently diagnosed with Parkinson's disease. Her healthcare provider feels she needs to take a MAO-B inhibitor to increase her dopamine level. The healthcare provider prescribes 50 mg of Xadago.

3. You explain to Mrs. Graham that she should restrict foods with tyramine. When she asks you to identify foods with tyramine, what are some foods that you list? (Check all that apply.)
   1. Aged cheeses
   2. Cured meats
   3. Melons
   4. Smoked meats
   5. Pickled foods
   6. Tea
   7. Soybeans
   8. Beer
   9. Wine
   10. Dried fruits

PRACTICE QUIZ

1. What is the composition of the central nervous system?
   a. Nerves extending from the spinal cord
   b. Organs, limbs, muscles, and blood vessels
   c. Brain and spinal cord
   d. Brain, heart, liver, lungs, and kidneys

2. What are the chemicals released from nerve endings that bind with subsequent nerves?
   a. Neurotransmitters
   b. Myelin
   c. Enzymes
   d. Epinephrine

3. The reduction of what chemical within the central nervous system causes Parkinson's disease?
   a. Substantia nigra
   b. Acetylcholine
   c. Dopamine
   d. Serotonin

4. When a patient diagnosed with Parkinson's disease develops cogwheel rigidity, what is the implication for the patient's movement?
   a. Facial features become masklike
   b. Arms and legs catch in stop-and-go movements
   c. Muscles become overly relaxed
   d. Hand tremors

5. Why will all Parkinson's disease patients eventually require dopamine?
   a. All other drug therapies wear off after age 70
   b. It is converted to natural dopamine.
   c. It reduces overproduction of dopamine caused by other drug therapies.
   d. It reduces symptoms of dyskinesia.

6. At what point are cholinesterase inhibitors no longer effective in the treatment of Alzheimer's disease?
   a. When the brain size shrinks and can no longer produce acetylcholinesterase
   b. When the number of neural transmitters sufficiently decrease
   c. When the patient's ability to swallow is impaired
   d. When there are fewer intact neurons available to make acetylcholine

7. What kinds of patient information does the Alzheimer's Disease Assessment Scale evaluate?
   a. Multiple organ functions
   b. Cognition, behavior, quality of life
   c. Chemical production within the central nervous system
   d. Muscle and respiratory fitness

8. Although antiepileptic drugs can reduce or prevent seizures, what are is at least one of their other uses?
   a. They can be used temporarily to reduce anxiety.
   b. They can be used to fight certain types of neural infections.
   c. They can be used to reduce muscle fatigue in patients with Parkinson's disease.
   d. They can be used to increase brain activity in late-stage patients with Alzheimer's disease.

9. Most of the newer antiepileptic drugs are used along with other drugs, which is referred to as what kind of drug therapy?
   a. Monotherapy
   b. Adjuvant therapy
   c. Multiagent neurotherapy
   d. Antigen therapy

10. What is one of the side-effects that is common to many of the antiepileptic drugs?
    a. Rash
    b. Increased sodium levels
    c. Folic acid deficiency
    d. Blurred or double vision

11. What is the most common form of multiple sclerosis?
    a. Relapsing-remitting MS
    b. Secondary progressive MS
    c. Primary progressive MS
    d. Progressive relapsing MS

12. What was originally the only type of drug therapy available for patients with multiple sclerosis?
    a. Biological response modifiers
    b. Corticosteroids
    c. Monoclonal antibodies
    d. Neurologic drugs

13. What are the rare adverse reactions of the drug riluzole, given to patients with ALS?
    a. Delusions and hallucinations
    b. Neutropenia, anemia, and kidney dysfunction
    c. Dyskinesia
    d. Insomnia

14. A patient is being given riluzole for treatment of ALS. How long will this drug prolong the patient's life?
    a. 6 months
    b. 1 year
    c. 3 months
    d. 6 years

15. Why is the extended release form of pyridostigmine given to patients who have weakness at night and upon awakening?
    a. Enhance patient safety from falls
    b. Prevent stomach distress
    c. Increase drowsiness so patient can sleep
    d. Avoid hypotension

11 Drugs for Mental Health

MULTIPLE CHOICE

Select the best answer for each of these following questions about mental health.

1. Which of the following is the best definition of mental illness?
   a. Mental illness results from genetic predispositions and drug or alcohol abuse.
   b. Mental illness is a condition that impacts a person's ability to think and also includes changes in behaviors and emotions.
   c. Mental illness is a condition defined by how an individual relates to environmental stressors and whether the behavior exhibited is considered clinically normal.
   d. Mental illness results from traumatic incidents and an individual's inability to process the experience in a mentally healthy way.

2. Along the continuum of mental health or mental illness, which of the following best indicates when an individual is experiencing mental illness?
   a. Experiencing and coping with stress to mild distress
   b. Increased use of food to cope with stress
   c. Mild or temporary impairment due to coping with distress
   d. Moodiness including tears and/or inappropriate behavior

3. According to the National Institute of Mental Health, approximately how many adults experience some degree of mental illness?
   a. 22%
   b. 4%
   c. 18% of women and 4% of men
   d. 18%

4. When a patient experiences sleep deprivation over an extended period of time, what are some of the more obvious impairments he or she might exhibit?
   a. Hand trembling, nervous tics
   b. Remembering, judgment, coordination
   c. Snoring, nausea, muscle pain
   d. Gregariousness, introversion, talkativeness

5. Which of the following diagnoses is associated with persons who have chronic or disabling anxiety?
   a. Insomnia
   b. Conduct disorder
   c. Attention-deficit disorder
   d. Social anxiety disorder

6. What is a general definition of psychosis?
   a. Loss of contact with reality
   b. Symptoms of delirium lasting more than 90 days
   c. Condition that is diagnosed such as schizophrenia or dementia
   d. Symptoms of delirium induced by alcohol or drugs

7. Which of the following is a common symptom of significant depression?
   a. Sadness triggered by the loss of a loved one
   b. Crying on a daily basis while at home or in the office
   c. Prolonged inability to perform activities of daily living
   d. Loss of interest in sex

8. Mood stabilizers are prescribed primarily for patients with what kind of illness?
   a. Bipolar illness
   b. Schizophrenia
   c. Depression
   d. Delirium

MATCHING

Match the chemical neurotransmitter on the right with the area affected on the left.

Areas Affected by Neurotransmitter

9. _____ Learning, movement, motivation, and drive

10. _____ Parasympathetic nervous system

11. _____ Sympathetic nervous system, alertness and arousal

12. _____ Sleep, appetite, pain, mood

13. _____ Inhibitory neurotransmitter, sleep, muscle tension

Neurotransmitters

A. Norepinephrine
B. Serotonin
C. Dopamine
D. Gamma-aminobutyric acid (GABA)
E. Acetylcholine

61

SELECT ALL THAT APPLY

For each of the drugs listed below, check all the statements that are true.

14. Benzodiazepines

_____ Used primarily for pregnant women

_____ Sedating-hypnotic drugs that depress the central nervous system

_____ High risk of dependency

_____ Enhance dopamine effects, leading to reduction in anxiety

15. Nonbenzodiazepine

_____ Makes the central nervous system less responsive to stimuli

_____ May be used to reduce anxiety

_____ Safe for use with patients who have liver impairment

16. Buspirone

_____ Reduces anxiety by affecting the serotonin and GABA neurotransmitters

_____ Decreases muscle tension, sweating, and rapid heart rate

_____ Sedation and high risk for physical dependence are possible

17. Typical antipsychotics

_____ Block dopamine receptors to treat symptoms such as hallucinations and delusions

_____ Can create pseudoparkinsonism

_____ May affect the body's ability to regulate core body temperature

_____ Adverse reactions can include neuroleptic malignant syndrome, characterized by an abnormally low body temperature

18. Atypical antipsychotics

_____ Used primarily for depression and anxiety

_____ May block dopamine receptors as well as some subtypes of serotonin

_____ Recommended for patients with psychosis from dementia

_____ Most common side effects are insomnia and drowsiness

_____ Clozapine is associated with decreased white blood cell count

_____ Weight loss is common

19. Selective serotonin reuptake inhibitors (SSRIs)

_____ Increase concentration of serotonin available to bind to dopamine receptors

_____ Sexual side effects are common in both men and women

_____ Increased risk of suicide

_____ Adverse effects include low sodium levels

_____ Safe for women who are pregnant or nursing

20. Serotonin norepinephrine reuptake inhibitors (SNRIs)

_____ Increase concentration of serotonin and norepinephrine neurotransmitters available to postsynaptic receptors

_____ Used for depression, fibromyalgia, and diabetic neuropathy

_____ Side effects include increased appetite

_____ Some patients experience increased sweating

_____ Adverse effects include nosebleeds

_____ Some patients can experience low sodium levels

21. Tricyclic antidepressants (TCAs)

_____ Have more side effects than SSRIs and SNRIs

_____ Reserved for individuals who do not respond to other treatments

_____ Used for patients with obsessive-compulsive disorder

_____ Can cause vision problems

_____ Can cause delirium in older patients with cognitive impairment

22. Monoamine oxidase inhibitors (MAOIs)

_____ MAOIs are enzymes that break down neurotransmitters

_____ Used to treat eating disorders

_____ Weight loss occurs in almost 10% of patients

_____ May cause hypotension if the patient ingests aged cheese and other foods and drinks containing tyramine

23. Mood stabilizers

_____ Lithium is used in short-term therapy of acute mania

_____ Lithium does not cause sedation or euphoria

_____ Lithium can cause mild weight gain

_____ Hand tremors are frequent

_____ Adverse reactions include hyperthyroidism

FILL IN THE BLANK

Patient and Family Education

24. Only take drugs for sleep if you have 5 to 6 hours available in order to avoid excessive _____.

25. Do not take a sedative with _____ or any other drug that depresses the central nervous system.

26. Nonbenzodiazepine drugs can cause you to be _____ active at night.

27. Avoid drinking _____ juice when taking benzodiazepines and nonbenzodiazepines.

28. Effects of drugs can decrease through use of _____ products and _____ beverages.

29. Suddenly stopping typical antipsychotics can result in nausea, dizziness, and _____.

30. Typical antipsychotics can affect your body's ability to adjust to changes in _____.

31. If you develop unusual muscle _____ while taking typical antipsychotics, contact your healthcare provider.

32. You can take most atypical antipsychotics with _____ to avoid GI upset.

33. Take SSRIs in the _____ to avoid insomnia.

34. St. John's wort can cause adverse effects if taken with _____.

35. Some patients have increased thoughts of _____ when first taking SSRIs and SNRIs.

36. Taking SNRIs during pregnancy can cause _____ abstinence syndrome in newborns.

37. It may take several _____ on SNRIs before you feel better.

38. TCAs can cause you to be more sensitive to _____, so wear protective clothing.

39. When taking TCAs, you should wear a medical alert _____.

40. The effects of MAO inhibitors can still be in your system for up to _____ weeks after discontinuing the drug.

41. Notify your healthcare provider if you experience a sudden _____ while taking MAO inhibitors.

42. You can mix the liquid version of lithium with _____ juices or other flavored drinks.

43. Avoid significant changes in your _____ and fluid intake.

44. Physical exertion can increase _____ and increase risk of lithium levels.

Chapter **11** **Drugs for Mental Health**

MATCHING

Match the drug on the left with the appropriate drug category on the right-hand side.

Drug Names

45. _____ Imipramine

46. _____ Estazolam

47. _____ Fluoxetine

48. _____ Venlafaxine

49. _____ Chlorpromazine

50. _____ Sertraline

51. _____ Aripiprazole

52. _____ Haloperidol

53. _____ Phenelzine

54. _____ Risperidone

55. _____ Zaleplon

56. _____ Lorazepam

57. _____ Lithium

58. _____ Bupropion

59. _____ Duloxetine

Drug Categories

A. Benzodiazepines
B. Nonbenzodiazepines
C. Typical antipsychotics
D. Atypical antipsychotics
E. Dopamine system stabilizers
F. Atypical antidepressants
G. Selective serotonin reuptake inhibitors
H. Serotonin and norepinephrine reuptake inhibitors
I. Tricyclic antidepressants
J. Monoamine oxidase inhibitors
K. Mood stabilizers

CASE STUDIES

Marcus Brooks is an 18-year-old man who has been suffering with depression for at least a year. His mother states he often stays in his room, does not socialize with friends, and is not doing well in school. He has a decreased appetite and is losing weight. He does not want to take antidepressants, but his mother is concerned and persuaded him to speak to a healthcare provider about his problem. After the assessment, Marcus was prescribed a SSRI antidepressant. To prevent noncompliance, it was explained to him that SSRIs are safer and more easily tolerated than other antidepressants.

1. Why is there an increased risk for when taking SSRIs during the first few months of treatment, especially for young adults and children? (Select the correct answer.)
   1. Hyperhidrosis
   2. Nosebleeds
   3. Suicidal ideation
   4. Elevated blood pressure

2. Marcus asks if he can stop the SSRIs anytime he wants if he does not like them. What do you explain to him? (Select all that apply.)
   1. There are many categories of antidepressants, so before stopping, discuss other alternative drugs with your healthcare provider.
   2. Some of the side effects that make you uncomfortable may go away after several weeks of taking the drug.
   3. Stopping the SSRI abruptly may cause ocular pressure leading to glaucoma.
   4. Sudden discontinuation of the SSRI may cause unpleasant withdrawal symptoms, so tapering is necessary.
   5. Discontinuing the SSRI may cause serotonin syndrome.
   6. Sexual side effects, such as lack of desire, inability to have an orgasm, or erectile dysfunction, can be discussed with the healthcare provider, who can suggest other drugs to help with those side effects.

Daisy Jones is 58 years old and for the last 6 months, has struggled with sleeping. As a consequence, she is having a difficult time performing throughout the day. After an examination, her healthcare provider prescribes 2 mg of Lunesta. You review what Ms. Jones should know about Lunesta before taking the drug.

3. What are some cautions Ms. Jones should be aware of before she begins taking Lunesta? (Select all that apply.)
    1. Do not drive or operate machinery while taking the drug.
    2. Defer making important decisions while taking the drug.
    3. Encourage Ms. Jones to take Lunesta with a cup of coffee.
    4. Let Ms. Jones know she may have a metallic taste in her mouth.
    5. Do not take Lunesta on an empty stomach.
    6. Make Ms. Jones aware not to take alcohol with Lunesta.
    7. Encourage Ms. Jones to only take Lunesta when she has sufficient time to sleep.
    8. Tell Ms. Jones to report any unusual agitation.
    9. If Lunesta is not sufficient to aid in sleep, combine it with an OTC drug.
    10. If necessary, take more than 1 dosage to help aid sleep.

4. After 3 months of taking Lunesta, Ms. Jones reports that she has gained excessive weight. What could be the possible reason?
    1. Lunesta causes weight gain.
    2. Ms. Jones may be sleepwalking and eating while on the drug.
    3. She has been sleeping later and not exercising since taking Lunesta.
    4. Ms. Jones is retaining water.

PRACTICE QUIZ

1. What is the main purpose of sedatives?
    a. To reduce anxiety in individuals who are unable to function due to stress
    b. To treat bipolar disease and reduce the symptoms that cause individuals to be anxious
    c. To promote sleep by changing signals in the central nervous system and reducing responses to stimulation
    d. To block neurotransmitters that are overactive and lead to hyperactivity in patients who are unable to sleep

2. Why is caffeine not recommended when taking either nonbenzodiazepines or benzodiazepines?
    a. Caffeine reduces the effectiveness of sedative drugs.
    b. Caffeine causes central nervous system depression, which deepens the sedative effect and can lead to death.
    c. Caffeine and sedatives combined can decrease the effectiveness of oral contraceptives.
    d. Caffeine can be used as an antidote for overdoses of sedatives.

3. Which disorder is not considered an anxiety disorder?
    a. Posttraumatic stress disorder
    b. Obsessive-compulsive disorder
    c. Panic disorder
    d. Bipolar disorder

4. For long-term mental health concerns, what are some of the best nonpharmacological therapies, other than counseling, for which you can provide information to your patient to assist in his or her recovery?
    a. Weight training, pet therapy, volunteering at a homeless shelter
    b. Vacation, spa days, socializing at a friendly tavern
    c. Mindfulness training, meditation, yoga
    d. Vegan diet, reading inspirational books, religious practice

5. Which of the following is a positive symptom of schizophrenia?
    a. Hallucinations
    b. Muscle rigidity
    c. Flat affect
    d. Cessation of delirium

6. Which of the following is a negative symptom of schizophrenia?
    a. Hallucinations
    b. Muscle rigidity
    c. Flat affect
    d. Cessation of delirium

7. What condition significantly contributes to the disease of schizophrenia?
    a. Overstimulation of dopamine
    b. Lack of serotonin
    c. Overstimulation of central nervous system
    d. Lack of norepinephrine

8. What is the main adverse effect to typical antipsychotic drugs?
    a. Drug dependence and possible addiction
    b. Extrapyramidal symptoms related to decrease in dopamine
    c. Greater rate of cognitive impairment and stroke risk
    d. Extreme fatigue due to increase in serotonin

65

9. While most extrapyramidal symptoms occur several days or weeks after beginning drug therapy, which one can occur after long-term use or even after the drug is discontinued?
   a. Akathisia
   b. Pseudoparkinsonism
   c. Acute dystonia
   d. Tardive dyskinesia

10. What is one of the advantages of taking atypical antipsychotics rather than typical antipsychotics?
    a. The chances of drug dependency are greatly reduced.
    b. They are recommended for patients with psychosis from dementia.
    c. They treat the negative as well as the positive symptoms common in some mental illnesses.
    d. They do not block dopamine receptors.

11. In addition to mental illnesses such as schizophrenia, what other disorders can be treated by dopamine system stabilizers?
    a. Sleep disorders
    b. Parkinson's disease
    c. Tourette's syndrome
    d. Epilepsy

12. Mild to moderate depression that lasts up to 2 years is labeled as what type of disorder?
    a. Mood disorder
    b. Dysthymic disorder
    c. Bipolar I disorder
    d. Chronic depression disorder

13. Which of the listed items can increase a patient's risk of serotonin syndrome?
    a. St. John's wort*
    b. Typical antipsychotic drugs
    c. NSAIDs
    d. Caffeinated beverages

14. Which tyramine-containing foods should not be ingested when a patient is taking monoamine oxidase inhibitors?
    a. Beef, salmon, dairy
    b. Cured or smoked meats, beer, wine, overripe fruits
    c. Foods containing gluten such as breads and pastas
    d. Overly processed foods such as cookies, chips, boxed foods

15. How do mood stabilizers work with patients diagnosed with bipolar disorder?
    a. Prevent the patient from becoming too depressed
    b. Eventually alleviate all symptoms over a period of time when supplemented with talk therapy
    c. Manage symptoms associated with both mania and depression
    d. Reduce the "highs" associated with the disorder to enable patient to function in most environments

12 Drugs for Pain Management

CROSSWORD PUZZLE

Identify the miscellaneous drug, based on the type of pain it most commonly relieves.

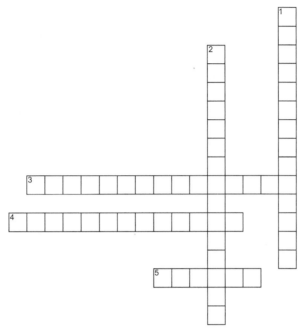

ACROSS

3. Reduces brain seizures and helps minimize pain from neuropathy and migraines
4. Manages mild to moderate pain and often used in place of aspirin.
5. Manages pain associated with inflammation, bone pain, cancer pain, and soft tissue trauma

DOWN

1. Improves long-term sadness and helps manage certain types of chronic pain such as neuropathy
2. Provides powerful anti-inflammatory actions

MATCHING

Match the types of pain management drugs with one of the four main categories. Each category can be selected more than once.

Pain Management Drugs

6. _____ Fentanyl

7. _____ Tylenol

8. _____ Pentazocine

9. _____ Buprenorphine

10. _____ Clonidine

11. _____ Hydrocodone

12. _____ Aspirin

13. _____ Tramadol

Categories

A. Opioid agonists
B. Opioid agonist-antagonists
C. Nonopioid centrally acting analgesics
D. Miscellaneous analgesics

67

FILL IN THE BLANK

Identify the type of pain (severe, moderate, mild) most frequently managed with each of the categories.

14. Opioid agonists such as morphine are used most often to manage _____ acute or chronic pain.

15. Opioid agonist-antagonist are used to manage _____ pain, primarily because there is a lower risk for addiction.

16. Nonopioid centrally acting analgesics blocks pain at the source and can also be used to manage _____ acute pain and lower blood pressure.

17. Miscellaneous analgesics can in some cases be purchased over the counter and are used to manage _____ pain. Some forms are able to reduce inflammation.

MATCHING

Match each of the following side effects and adverse reactions with a specific type of drug.

Side Effect and/or Adverse Reaction

18. _____ Elevation of blood pressure

19. _____ Increased risk for bleeding

20. _____ Cardiac dysrhythmias

21. _____ Hypotension

22. _____ High does for prolonged periods can cause liver damage

23. _____ Sleepiness, constipation, respiratory depression

24. _____ Blurred vision, dizziness, urinary retention

25. _____ Seizures

Drug

A. Morphine
B. Pentazocine
C. Buprenorphine
D. Clonidine
E. Tramadol
F. Acetaminophen
G. NSAIDs
H. Cyclobenzaprine

SHORT ANSWERS

Write a brief description of how you would manage each of the following situations.

26. Mrs. Smith has been receiving morphine for several days. What is one question you would ask her to ensure she will not experience further discomfort?

27. Mr. Jones has been given a prescription for an opioid and will be cared for by his wife. You are providing her with information for his care. How can she help prevent dizziness and falling?

28. Ms. Washington has been prescribed tramadol for a back injury. What is an important question to ask her before she begins this medication?

29. After administering Mr. Reyes first dose of cyclobenzaprine, what should you assess on an hourly basis?

CASE STUDIES

Marvin Ford, a 62-year-old man, has been diagnosed with diabetes type 2. He is obese and lives a sedentary lifestyle. He presents with neuropathic pain in his feet. He states he has pain daily and the pain is often accompanied by numbness, a burning sensation, and a tingling feeling, especially when he walks. His healthcare provider prescribes the antidepressant sertraline (Zoloft) for Mr. Ford.

1. How does an antidepressant help with chronic pain? (Choose the correct answer.)
    1. Antidepressants can help with chronic pain by increasing natural opioids.
    2. Antidepressants increase the amount of insulin produced.
    3. Antidepressants help patients to avoid thinking about pain.
    4. Antidepressants help patients to lose weight and increase activity level, thereby reducing neuropathic pain.

2. What other class of nonopioid drugs can relieve chronic pain? (Choose the correct answer.)
    1. Antihistamines
    2. Anticholinergics
    3. Anticonvulsives
    4. Antifungals

Selma Reed is a 76-year-old woman who has stage 4 peritoneal cancer and is experiencing occasional bouts of intense pain. Her healthcare provider has prescribed 2 mg of hydromorphone to be taken every 4 hours, as needed for pain.

3. What types of health conditions do you warn the healthcare provider about Mrs. Reed takes the drug? (Select all that apply.)
    1. Asthma
    2. Slowed breathing
    3. Osteoarthritis
    4. COPD
    5. Autoimmune disease
    6. Head injury
    7. Kyphoscoliosis
    8. History of DVTs

4. When Mrs. Reed first begins taking the drug, what should you do to ensure safety?
    1. Offer Mrs. Reed oxygen if she begins having trouble breathing.
    2. Assess respiratory rate and pulse oximetry frequently.
    3. Measure temperature and blood pressure every 2 hours.
    4. Check frequently to see if the pain improves.

PRACTICE QUIZ

1. How do you assess whether a patient is experiencing pain?
    a. By observing his or her body movements
    b. By asking the patient to identify whether he or she is in pain
    c. Based on when the patient last received a prescribed dosage of pain relief medication
    d. By monitoring vital signs to determine if there are significant changes

2. Identify which of the following situations is likely acute (A) or chronic (C) pain.
    a. _____ Osteoarthritis of the knee
    b. _____ Urinary tract infection
    c. _____ Broken bone
    d. _____ Chemo-induced peripheral neuropathy

3. Which of the following conditions is most likely to increase a patient's perception of pain?
    a. A stroke that destroys a part of the brain
    b. Anxiety and/or depression
    c. A quiet, relaxing environment
    d. Regular use of alternative therapies such as meditation

69

4. Identify which of the following is not an Agency for Healthcare Research and Quality principle for pain management.
   a. Use of pain intensity scales in order to assess pain systematically
   b. Making sure to ask about pain on a regular basis
   c. Not trusting the patient or family regarding their perceptions or opinions regarding pain
   d. Allowing patients to manage their pain management as much as possible

5. You have a patient still in pain but cannot reach the healthcare provider for a prescription. There are several nondrug options that you can utilize instead. Which of the following, however, would _not_ be a suitable nondrug therapy for pain relief?
   a. Ice or cold compresses
   b. Six ounces of red wine or 1 ounce of liquor
   c. Exercise
   d. Acupuncture

6. Analgesics are a category of drug developed specifically to reduce pain. How do these drugs work when administered to a patient who is in pain?
   a. They change the patient's perception of pain or reduction of painful stimulation at its source.
   b. They calm the patient to an extent where he or she does not register any pain
   c. They address the source of the actual pain by reducing inflammation.
   d. They create a sense of euphoria in the patient so that he or she forgets about the pain.

7. Opioids are an analgesic drug used to manage severe pain. Natural opioids are derived from opium. What are synthetic opioids, such as hydrocodone and oxycodone, made from?
   a. Heroin
   b. Morphine
   c. Coca plant
   d. Poppy plant

8. What is the reason all opioids, both natural and synthetic, are labeled _high-alert drugs_?
   a. They must be kept under lock and key to prevent theft because of their cost.
   b. Patients can occasionally become overly excited when taking opioids.
   c. Allergic reactions are frequent with their use.
   d. They have an increased risk for causing patient harm.

9. Morphine is the drug by which all other pain-management drugs are compared for effectiveness. Which drug from the list below is actually stronger than morphine?
   a. Codeine
   b. Hydrocodone
   c. Dilaudid
   d. Oxycodone

10. If a patient has a strong adverse reaction or overdose after taking an opioid agonist, such as morphine, how can the effects be reversed?
    a. Induce vomiting by administering an emetic.
    b. Administer an opioid antagonist such as naloxone.
    c. Inject fentanyl intramuscularly or subcutaneously.
    d. Keep the patient awake and help them move as much as possible until effects diminish.

11. Opioid agonist-antagonists are used for less severe pain and are less addictive than opioid agonists, but they can be responsible for causing which of the following reactions?
    a. Severe cardiac reactions
    b. Severe diarrhea
    c. Severe respiratory reactions
    d. Severe dehydration

12. How do nonopioid centrally acting analgesics, such as clonidine and tramadol, help manage pain?
    a. Interacting with opioid receptors
    b. Stimulating the endorphins
    c. Blocking activity in the central nervous system
    d. Enhancing a feeling of euphoria

13. Which drug can lead to hypotension through dilation of blood vessels?
    a. Tramadol
    b. Butorphanol
    c. OxyContin
    d. Clonidine

14. Miscellaneous analgesics are used to treat less severe pain and unlike opioids can reduce symptoms of pain by which of the following methods?
    a. Increasing the production of endorphins to promote healing
    b. Reducing the symptoms of inflammation by helping stop tissue production of the chemical of inflammation
    c. Raising blood pressure to provide more blood flow to sites that are damaged
    d. Preventing dehydration

15. Which of the following drugs is used to reduce pain from muscular contractions or spasms?
    a. Cyclobenzaprine
    b. Nabumetone
    c. Prednisone
    d. Acetaminophen

13 Drugs for Inflammation, Arthritis, and Gout

IDENTIFYING TYPES OF DRUGS

Match the drug name with the category of drugs.

Drugs

1. _____ Aspirin

2. _____ Prednisone

3. _____ Etanercept

4. _____ Triamcinolone

5. _____ Nabumetone

6. _____ Meloxicam

7. _____ Allopurinol

8. _____ Celecoxib

9. _____ Adalimumab

10. _____ Dexamethasone

Drug Categories

A. Cyclooxygenase 1 and 2 (COX-1) inhibitors (nonselective NSAIDs)
B. Cyclooxygenase 2 (COX-2) inhibitors (selective NSAIDs)
C. Corticosteroids
D. Disease-modifying antirheumatic drugs
E. Uric acid synthesis inhibitors

MULTIPLE SELECTION

Identify all the statements that are applicable for each of the drug categories.

11. Nonsteroidal anti-inflammatory drugs (NSAIDs)

_____ Rapidly increase production of one or more inflammatory mediators

_____ COX-1 inhibitor drugs block both COX-1 and COX-2 enzymes when inflammation occurs within the body

_____ NSAIDs are the first-line therapy against illnesses associated with pain and/or fever

_____ NSAIDs are not used for any type of arthritis

_____ Monitor patients who take aspirin for bleeding

Adverse reactions to NSAIDs

_____ Mild to serious allergic reactions

_____ Severe GI distress

_____ Myocardial infarction and stroke

_____ Reye's syndrome in elderly

12. Corticosteroids

_____ Manage severe or chronic inflammation

_____ Used in any condition that could lead to tissue damage

_____ Slow production of red blood cells

_____ Can only be administered orally

Adverse reactions to corticosteroids

_____ Adrenal glands quit producing cortisol

_____ Increased number of white blood cells

_____ Delirium or extreme behavior changes

_____ Respiratory failure

13. Disease-modifying antirheumatic drugs (DMARDs)

_____ Reduce tissue damage of the inflammatory disease process by inhibiting cortisol

_____ Inhibit inflammatory mediator tumor necrosis factor (TNF)

_____ Tissue damage is reduced, but pain is not relieved, so patients require additional drugs for relieving pain and improving physical function

_____ DMARDs are used in the treatment of chronic inflammatory diseases that involve tissue destruction caused by excessive inflammatory mediators

Adverse Reactions to DMARDs

_____ Reduced immune response, increasing risk for infections

_____ Heart failure

14. Antigout drugs

_____ Reduce the amount of enzymes that convert purines in protein into uric acid

_____ To prevent gout, these drugs must be taken daily

_____ Lower uric acid levels that occur during rapid cell destruction

Adverse reactions to antigout drugs

_____ Increased risk of infection

_____ Gallstones

_____ Liver failure

PATIENT & FAMILY TEACHING

Provide a short answer to each of the following questions.

Teaching Patients and Families About NSAIDs

15. Why should NSAIDs be taken with a full glass of water?

_____

16. Contact your healthcare provider if you experience any of the following symptoms.

_____

17. How many glasses of water a day should you drink?

_____

Teaching Patients and Families About Corticosteroids

18. Why could heavy smoking be a problem?

_____

19. What are at least three symptoms that could indicate a life-threatening problem with the patient's adrenal glands?

_____

20. Why should the patient eat a diet rich in potassium and low in sodium?

_____

21. What are at least three symptoms of hypokalemia (decreased potassium in the blood)?

_____

22. What are at least three symptoms indicating the patient may be having problems with the liver?

_____

23. What are at least three symptoms indicating the patient may have an infection?

_____

24. What should patients avoid until contacting their healthcare providers while taking DMARDs?

_____

Teaching Patients and Families About Antigout Drugs

25. How should the patient take allopurinol?

_____

26. How much liquid should the patient drink?

_____

27. What types of foods should the patient avoid?

_____

28. Which antigout drug is not impacted by meals or antacids?

_____

CASE STUDIES

Mrs. Dorothy Stubbins, a 72-year-old female, has been diagnosed with rheumatoid arthritis. She has been treated by her primary care doctor for several years. Her condition has been getting worse and the medications used have not been effective. Mrs. Stubbins's primary care doctor referred her to a rheumatologist to discuss trying disease-modifying antirheumatic drugs (DMARDs) to prevent or limit bone loss.

1. What questions are necessary for Mrs. Stubbins's assessment before beginning DMARDs? (Select all that apply.)
   1. Ask her to list every drug she is currently taking.
   2. Check for the presence of any prior allergy to aspirin or other NSAIDs, history of asthma, blood disorders, GI problems or ulcer disease, or other liver or kidney problems.
   3. Ask about symptoms of infection such as fever, cough, foul-smelling drainage, pain or burning on urination, and general malaise.
   4. Find out if she has had any recent exposure to people who are ill.
   5. Determine whether she has received an immunization within the past month.
   6. Check for any redness around a wound or other open skin area.
   7. All patients must be tested for tuberculosis before starting DMARDs.
   8. Always ask patients about whether they have a current infection or have had any of these infections in the past: tuberculosis, hepatitis, shingles, HIV infection, pneumocystis pneumonia, or any type of opportunistic infection.

2. How do DMARDs reduce the progression and tissue destruction of Mrs. Stubbins's inflammatory disease process, especially rheumatoid arthritis?
   1. By preventing or limiting inflammation by slowing or stopping all known pathways of inflammatory cytokine production
   2. By preventing or limiting the tissue and blood vessel responses to injury by slowing the production of one or more inflammatory mediators
   3. By inhibiting tumor necrosis factor (TNF)
   4. By preventing or limiting the tissue and blood vessel responses to injury or invasion

73

George Stevens, a 58-year-old man suffers from mild osteoarthritis. He particularly has trouble with his knees. As his job involves squatting and kneeling, it becomes frequently uncomfortable. Because his pain is not severe, his healthcare provider recommends he begin taking aspirin for the pain.

3. What are some important recommendations you should make to Mr. Stevens to ensure he is safe while taking aspirin? (Select all that apply.)
   1. Stop taking aspirin at least 1 week before any dental or surgical procedures.
   2. Limit leafy green vegetables and beans from his diet.
   3. Report any signs of blood in the stool.
   4. Do not drink caffeinated beverages.
   5. Do not take aspirin if taking warfarin.
   6. Ensure he is vaccinated from influenza.
   7. Weigh himself at least twice a week.
   8. It is best to take aspirin with food.

PRACTICE QUIZ

1. What are the five major symptoms of inflammation?
   a. Nausea, fever, warmth, swelling, loss of function
   b. Pain, redness, warmth, swelling, loss of function
   c. Nausea, redness, warmth, swelling, loss of function
   d. Pain, redness, warmth, swelling, loss of muscle control

2. How do inflammatory responses within the body help injured tissue regain function?
   a. Trigger swelling around damaged joints to protect underlying tissue
   b. Prevent autoimmune diseases from developing
   c. Stimulate healthy cell growth to replace dead or damaged cells
   d. Block scar tissue development

3. What is one condition that can occur if inflammation does not go away when no longer needed or occurs when there is no injury?
   a. Serious and painful tissue damage
   b. Life-threatening infections
   c. Loss of muscle control in the affected area
   d. The inflammatory response can spread to other areas within the body.

4. Why is it important to monitor patients who are taking anti-inflammatory drugs?
   a. It is only necessary to monitor patients who are taking anti-inflammatory drugs on a long-term basis.
   b. Taking anti-inflammatory drugs incorrectly can lead to permanent damage to the heart and liver.
   c. Development of scar tissue while taking drugs can prevent tissue from healing.
   d. There are adverse reactions to all anti-inflammatory drugs.

5. Why do COX-1 inhibitors, such as aspirin, cause more side effects than COX-2 inhibitors?
   a. COX-1 inhibitors block the cellular COX-1, which is protective, as well as inflammation associated with COX-2.
   b. COX-1 inhibitors block white blood cells necessary for healing the inflammation.
   c. COX-1 inhibitors, unlike COX-2 inhibitors, increase bleeding risks for patients taking anticoagulant.
   d. COX-1 inhibitors frequently lead to overdoses due to their availability as over-the-counter drugs.

6. When taking a history of a patient who has just suffered an injury leading to inflammation, what question should you be certain to include to ensure your patient's safety?
   a. Ask whether the patient can safely walk on his own or if he needs assistance
   b. Ask the patient if he is taking any over-the-counter drugs, including aspirin, on a regular basis
   c. Ask the patient is he prone to injuries or if this was a first time
   d. Ask the patient if he is taking any pain-relieving drugs obtained illegally

7. How do corticosteroid drugs prevent or limit inflammation?
   a. Inhibit cortisol hormone secreted by the adrenal gland
   b. Increase production of white blood cells in the bone marrow
   c. Slow or stop all known pathways of inflammatory cytokine production*
   d. Allow COX-1 and COX-2 enzymes to produce inflammatory mediators

8. Which of the conditions listed below are not treated by corticosteroids?
   a. Severe asthma
   b. Atrial fibrillation
   c. Systemic lupus erythematosus
   d. Acute adrenal emergencies

9. Why is it necessary for the patient to taper the dose of corticosteroids when discontinuing their use?
   a. Tapering lowers risk of infection as white blood cell production increases.
   b. Tapering allows the adrenal glands to begin producing sufficient cortisol again.
   c. Tapering prevents adverse effects such as delirium or mania.
   d. Tapering lowers risk of developing Cushing syndrome.

10. When assessing a patient prior to corticosteroid drug therapy, what is one of the most important conditions you need to identify?
    a. Ensure the patient does not have stomach issues, as GI bleeding could occur
    b. Ensure the patient is able to take the drug as prescribed, as missed dosages and discontinuing the drug can have severe consequences
    c. Ensure the patient does not have any infections, as corticosteroids can reduce immunity
    d. Ensure the patient is accurate regarding all prescribed and over-the-counter drugs he or she is currently taking

11. How do DMARDs reduce the progression of tissue destruction in inflammatory diseases?
    a. Prevent production of cortisol
    b. Inhibit tumor necrosis factor (TNF)
    c. Increase blood flow in damaged areas
    d. Reduce pain significantly, allowing for physical therapy

12. Why do patients taking DMARDs have a risk for developing anemia and an increased risk for bleeding?
    a. Thinning of skin increases the chances of bleeding and blood loss and consequently anemia.
    b. Frequent inactivity and nausea lead to weakness and lack of nutrients entering the body.
    c. Minerals are used in tissue repair and therefore are not available to protect the patient from other conditions, such as anemia.
    d. These drugs reduce bone marrow production of red blood cells and platelets

13. What must patients be tested for before starting a DMARD?
    a. Hepatitis C
    b. HIV
    c. Tuberculosis
    d. Emphysema

14. What lifestyle changes can 10% of persons diagnosed with gout make to control the disease?
    a. Eat little to no shellfish, specific other fish, red and organ meats, pork, beer, and wine
    b. Perform an hour of moderate exercise on a daily basis
    c. Remove all dairy, wheat, and sugar from the diet
    d. Do weight training three times per week

15. Which of the following statements describe how gout affects the body?
    a. Reactions to proteins within the blood create joint inflammation
    b. The kidneys are unable to efficiently eliminate urine and excess fluid causes swelling in joints
    c. Increase of uric acid crystals are deposited into the joints
    d. Swelling in joints due to leaking of fluid from capillaries

14 Drugs for Gastrointestinal Problems

KEY TERMS

Match the term to the correct definition

Definitions

1. _____ A category of drugs used to help neutralize gastric acid and reduce symptoms of indigestion and heartburn

2. _____ A category of drugs used to prevent and treat nausea and vomiting

3. _____ Drugs that reduce or stop loose, watery stools and help to restore normal bowel movements

4. _____ Drugs that are either natural or synthetic forms of THC that reduce nausea and vomiting by binding to both cannabinoid receptors in the chemoreceptor trigger zone (CTZ) and by preventing serotonin 5-HT$_3$ from binding to its receptors in the CTZ

5. _____ A class of drugs that protect the lining of the stomach and prevent further damage

6. _____ A class of drugs that inhibit the binding of histamine to H$_2$-receptors on the parietal cells in the stomach, thereby decreasing gastric acid secretions

7. _____ A class of drugs that promote bowel movements by stimulating peristalsis, increasing the bulk of the stool, or by softening the stool

8. _____ A class of antidiarrheal drugs that reduce GI motility and increase the ability of the intestine to absorb water

9. _____ A type of antiemetic drug that reduces nausea and vomiting by blocking dopamine receptors in the CTZ

10. _____ A class of drugs that increase contraction of the upper GI tract including the stomach and the small intestines to move contents more quickly through the tract by blocking dopamine 2 receptors in the CTZ and the intestinal tract

11. _____ A class of drugs that bind to the proton pump of the parietal cells in the stomach, which blocks acid secretion into the stomach

12. _____ A class of antiemetic drugs that reduce or halt nausea and vomiting by blocking (5-HT$_3$) receptors in the intestinal tract and the CTZ so serotonin cannot activate these receptors

13. _____ A class of antiemetic drugs that block the substance P/neurokinin$_1$ (NK$_1$) receptors in the CTZ, preventing the substance P and neurokinin that are released from cells exposed to chemotherapy and damage in surgery from binding to and triggering the CTZ

Terms

A. substance P/neurokinin$_1$ (NK$_1$) receptor antagonists
B. serotonin (5-HT$_3$) receptor antagonists
C. proton pump inhibitors
D. promotility drugs
E. antiemetic
F. antidiarrheal
G. antacids
H. phenothiazines
I. opioid agonists
J. laxatives
K. histamine H$_2$-receptor antagonists
L. cytoprotective drugs
M. cannabinoids

Chapter **14** **Drugs for Gastrointestinal Problems**

14. Complete the table.

NAME	ACTIONS	SIDE EFFECTS	ADVERSE EFFECTS
Serotonin (5-HT$_3$) receptor antagonists	Antiemetic drugs that reduce or halt nausea and vomiting by blocking (5-HT$_3$) receptors in the intestinal tract and the CTZ so serotonin cannot activate these receptors.	_____ _____ _____ _____ _____ _____ _____ _____	_____ _____ _____ _____ _____ _____ _____ _____
Substance P/neurokinin$_1$ (NK$_1$) receptor antagonists	_____ _____ _____ _____ _____ _____	Fatigue, diarrhea, head-ache and dizziness. The patient may experience mild hiccups, flatulence, and sweating.	_____ _____ _____ _____ _____
_____	Antiemetic drug that reduces nausea and vomiting by blocking dopamine (D$_2$) receptors in the CTZ of the brain. Approved to reduce nausea and vomiting from many problems except morning sickness associated with pregnancy.	_____ _____ _____ _____ _____ _____ _____ _____ _____ _____	Tardive dyskinesia, acute dystonia, and even neuroleptic malignant syndrome. Blood abnor-malities are possible. Patients with cardio-vascular disease can experience angina, tachy-cardia, and/or orthostatic hypotension.

NAME	ACTIONS	SIDE EFFECTS	ADVERSE EFFECTS
Cannabinoids	Drugs that are either natural or synthetic forms of THC that reduce nausea and vomiting by binding to both cannabinoid receptors in the CTZ and by preventing serotonin 5-HT$_3$ from binding to its receptors in the CTZ.	_____ _____ _____ _____ _____ _____ _____ _____ _____ _____	_____ _____ _____ _____ _____ _____ _____ _____ _____ _____
Promotility drugs	_____ _____ _____ _____ _____ _____ _____ _____ _____ _____ _____ _____ _____ _____	_____ _____ _____ _____ _____ _____ _____ _____ _____ _____ _____ _____ _____ _____	Can cause depression and even suicidal ideation, seizures, blood disorders, cardiac dysrhythmias, and heart failure. Symptoms similar to Parkinson's disease include tremor, bradykinesia, and mask-like facies. Severe adverse effects include *tardive dyskinesia, akathisia,* and *acute dystonia.*

TEACHING PATIENTS AND FAMILIES ABOUT ANTIEMETIC AND PROMOTILITY DRUGS

Fill in the blank for each of the topics below that describe the type of information patients and their families need to be aware of when taking antiemetic and promotility drugs.

15. Tell the pharmacist or your healthcare provider about any other _____ or prescribed drugs you are taking in order to avoid _____.

16. Avoid driving, operating any machinery, or _____ while taking antiemetic drugs because they may impair your judgment and _____.

17. It is best to take the antiemetic drug for nausea rather than waiting until after you have had an _____.

18. Do not use any alcohol or drugs with _____ while taking antiemetics.

19. If you are taking the oral solution of _____, avoid shaking the mixture. You can gently swirl and turn over the measuring cup or syringe.

20. Tell patients to _____ if they experience dizziness when taking phenothiazines.

Chapter **14** **Drugs for Gastrointestinal Problems**

21. Phenothiazines can decrease your ability to _____ and patients may become more sensitive to the sun. Advise patients to avoid _____ and _____.

22. Patients taking phenothiazines should contact their healthcare provider immediately if they experience any muscle spasm (particularly of the neck muscles); involuntary movements of the _____, _____, _____; or any unusual restlessness.

23. Patients should be taught to contact their healthcare provider immediately if they experience _____ or _____ when taking promotility drugs.

24. An increase of _____, _____, or _____ could be a sign of a more serious illness when taking promotility drugs and the patient should report it to their healthcare provider.

25. Some men may experience _____ or _____; some women may experience _____. These are generally reversible within a few weeks to a few months.

DRUGS FOR PEPTIC ULCER DISEASE AND GASTROESOPHAGEAL REFLUX DISEASE

Match the drug to the correct action, side effect, and adverse effect. Some answers will be used more than once.

Correct Actions, Side Effects, and Adverse Effects

Drugs

A. Antacids
B. Histamine H_2-receptor antagonists
C. Proton pump inhibitors (PPIs)
D. Cytoprotective drugs

26. _____ protect the lining of the stomach and protects it from further damage.

27. _____ Magnesium-based versions of this drug are usually related to hypermagnesemia, low blood pressure and low heart rate. Calcium-containing versions can cause bone pain, kidney stones, and in severe cases, cardiac dysrhythmias. Aluminum-containing versions can cause mood changes, confusion, osteoporosis, and hypercalcemia.

28. _____ bind to the H_2 receptor in the stomach cells, leading to a decrease in production of basal and nighttime gastric acid. They also decrease the amount of gastric acid released with meals and with substances such as caffeine.

29. _____ Side effects include headache, mild abdominal pain, nausea, and vomiting, flatulence, diarrhea or constipation, and increased sensitivity to light. Less common side effects include dizziness, anxiety, or mild rash.

30. _____ are drugs that neutralize hydrochloric acid (HCl) and increase gastric pH, which in turn reduces gastric irritation. They provide only temporary relief.

31. _____ Adverse reactions are rare and include severe allergic reactions, a variety of blood disorders, and cardiac dysrhythmias. While the reason is not fully known, patients may also be at risk for pneumonia.

32. _____ help heal gastric ulcers and reduce symptoms of GERD by stopping the acid secretory pump that is located within the gastric parietal cell membrane, therefore reducing the amount of acid secreted into the stomach.

33. _____ headache, nausea, diarrhea or constipation, and mild abdominal pain. Some patients may have mental status changes, including confusion, anxiety, or depression.

34. _____ Brands with magnesium can cause diarrhea; brands with calcium or aluminum can cause constipation. Other side effects include loss of appetite, frequent burping, nausea and vomiting, fatigue, and weight loss or depression.

35. _____ severe allergic reactions, pancreatitis, and blood abnormalities, including thrombocytopenia and hemolytic anemia. May have increased risk for osteoporosis and bone fracture with long-term use.

TEACHING PATIENTS AND FAMILIES ABOUT DRUGS FOR PEPTIC ULCER DISEASE AND GASTROESOPHEGAL REFLUX

Indicate which class of drugs matches the description of important information to teach patients and families. Some descriptions may have more than one answer.

Patient Information

36. _____ Wear sunscreen and protective clothing because your skin may be more sensitive to light.

37. _____ These drugs do not cure ulcers, but they do reduce acid in your stomach so that the ulcer can heal.

38. _____ These drugs are for temporary relief. If symptoms persist after two weeks or after completing a prescribed amount, contact your healthcare provider.

39. _____ Take the drug 1 hour after meals and before bedtime.

40. _____ Ask your family members to observe you for any changes in mental status, such as confusion or anxiety and depression.

41. _____ Once-a-day dosing of this drug is best taken at bedtime to reduce symptoms of acid reflux at night.

42. _____ These neutralize gastric acids and are typically most beneficial if given between meals and at bedtime.

43. _____ Do not drive or operate heavy machinery until you see how the drug affects you.

44. _____ Diarrhea or constipation are common side effects. Contact your healthcare provider if severe.

45. _____ If this drug is in chewable form, chew completely and follow with a glass of water. If liquid, be sure to shake well.

46. _____ Avoid driving or using heavy machinery while using this drug, as it may cause dizziness.

47. _____ Avoid cigarette smoking because it increases gastric acid production and can decrease the effectiveness of this drug.

48. _____ If you are taking other drugs, it is usually best to take them 1 hour before or 2 hours after taking this drug.

Class of Drugs

A. Antacids
H. Histamine H_2-receptor antagonists
P. Proton pump inhibitors (PPIs)

DRUGS FOR CONSTIPATION AND DIARRHEA

Laxatives

Fill in the blanks for each topic below that describes the uses, side effects, and adverse effects for patients using laxatives.

49. Laxatives are a class of drugs that promote bowel movements by stimulating _____, increasing the

_____ of the _____, or by _____ the _____.

50. Laxatives are generally for _____ but are also used for cleansing the bowel before an _____,

_____, or _____ procedure.

51. Describe how each type of laxative works to help relieve constipation:
    a. *Bulk-forming laxatives*

    _____

    _____

    _____

    _____

    b. *Lubricant laxatives*

    _____

    _____

    _____

    _____

    c. *Stool softeners*

    _____

    _____

    _____

    _____

    d. *Osmotic laxatives*

    _____

    _____

    _____

    e. *Stimulant* or irritant laxatives

    _____

    _____

    _____

    _____

52. The most common side effects of laxatives are GI symptoms such as _____,

    _____, _____, and _____.

Match the type of laxative that can cause the following adverse reactions.

Adverse Reactions

Laxatives

53. _____ Rarely, a condition called *lipid pneumonia* can occur by inhalation of fat-containing substances like mineral oil.

54. _____ Can produce and fluid and electrolyte disturbance if used daily or in patients with renal or cardiac impairment.

55. _____ May produce decreased absorption of nutrients and fat-soluble vitamins.

56. _____ Inhaling the psyllium dust particles can cause hypersensitivity reactions.

57. _____ Patients who do not take the drugs with enough water (need at least 8-12 ounces of fluid) are at risk for esophageal obstruction. Swelling of the throat or choking might occur.

58. _____ Severe allergic reactions are possible.

59. _____ May produce muscle weakness (following excessive use of laxatives), dermatitis, pruritus, alkalosis, and electrolyte imbalance (with excessive use).

A. Bulk-forming laxatives
B. Stool softeners
C. Lubricants
D. Osmotic laxatives
E. Stimulant laxatives

TEACHING PATIENTS AND FAMILIES ABOUT LAXATIVES

Fill in the blanks for the topics below that describe important information to teach patients and families about laxative use.

60. Most laxatives are recommended for _____ use only. Contact your healthcare provider if you require laxatives on a regular basis or do not have relief with over-the-counter drugs.

61. Some laxatives are high in _____ or in _____. Make sure to read the labels carefully if you are on a special diet.

62. Laxatives are not a substitute for good bowel habits, including _____ activity and a diet that includes high-fiber foods such as _____, _____, and _____.

63. Many types of drugs increase the risk of _____. If you are taking a drug that causes _____, contact your healthcare provider to determine the best type of laxative for you.

64. Never take a laxative to treat _____ _____ _____ because the drug may make conditions worse.

65. The onset of action of laxatives varies according to the specific drug category. These drugs can work in as short a period of time as an _____ or as long as _____. Knowing the expected onset will help you plan.

ANTIDIARRHEALS

Fill in the blanks for each topic below that describes the uses, side effects and adverse effects of antidiarrheals.

66. Antidiarrheals are drugs that reduce or stop _____, _____ _____, and help to restore normal bowel movements.

67. Three general drug classes are used to treat these problems: _____, _____ or _____.

68. Anticholinergics reduce GI tract _____ and intestinal _____, _____ production, and _____ motility and thus reduce the associated pain.

69. The antispasmodic drugs reduce _____ in the GI tract. This causes decreased cramping, bloating, and diarrhea.

70. Opioid agonists are effective for diarrhea but do not have the _____ or other opioid-like effects. They do, however, reduce GI motility and increase the ability of the intestine to absorb water. Stools then increase bulk and the patient loses fewer fluids and _____.

71. A fourth drug for diarrhea is _____. While the action is not fully understood, this drug may prevent the attachment of certain organisms to the intestinal _____ and provide a protective coating. It is used to treat nonspecific diarrhea and diarrhea caused by _____. It is also used to prevent _____ diarrhea.

72. The most common side effects of antidiarrheals include _____,_____, and _____. Other possible side effects may be dizziness or drowsiness.

73. _____ have many drug interactions that can cause adverse reactions. _____ taken with other opioid drugs can increase the opioid effect.

74. List at least three important topics that are important information to teach patients and families about antidiarrheals.

    1. _____
    _____

    2. _____
    _____

    3. _____
    _____

CASE STUDY

Mr. Wallace Higgins is an 87-year-old-man who has been diagnosed with hypertension and diabetes type II. He has been on medication for both diseases for several years. He is on a low sodium and low sugar diet. Recently, he came to the clinic presenting with severe constipation. He said he had been taking an over-the-counter laxative for six months at least three times a week.

1. What should you teach Mr. Higgins about over-the-counter laxatives? (Choose the correct answer.)
    1. When taking laxatives, Mr. Higgins should avoid high-fiber foods as they will increase the effect of the laxative.
    2. Many laxatives are high in sodium and sugar.
    3. Fluids should be avoided when taking bulk-forming laxatives as they interfere with the bulk-forming function.
    4. Exercise should be avoided when taking laxatives as movement causes an increase in the need for laxatives.

2. Mr. Higgins asks if it is okay that he uses a laxative often. How do you answer him?
    1. Laxatives are meant for short-term use only.
    2. Some of Mr. Higgins's other prescriptions cause constipation, so he should be using laxatives regularly to counteract the effect of the other drugs he takes.
    3. Laxatives should not be taken daily, but three times a week is acceptable.
    4. Mr. Higgins can use a laxative that often if he also follows his low sodium and low sugar diet.

Joan Perkins is a 45-year-old woman with early stage breast cancer. She is continuously nauseous and has been unable to keep down food or beverages. Her healthcare provider has tried a series of antiemetics but has been unable to find an adequate combination of drugs to reduce Ms. Perkins's nausea. As a last resort, she prescribes cannabinoids.

3. Ms. Perkins will receive liquid-filled capsules. How is her dosage individualized?
    1. Dosage is based on age.
    2. Dosage is based on how much is needed to stop the nausea.
    3. Dosage is based on what other drugs the patient is taking.
    4. Dosage is based on body surface area.

4. What should you advise Ms. Perkins to avoid while taking cannabinoids? (Select all that apply.)
    1. Alcohol
    2. Coffee
    3. NSAIDs
    4. Dairy products
    5. Central nervous system depressants
    6. Antacids high in sodium
    7. Illegal drugs
    8. OTC CBD products

84

1. What issues are patients at most risk for when experiencing nausea and vomiting?
   a. Dizziness, drowsiness and mental confusion
   b. Dehydration, weight loss and electrolyte imbalance
   c. Swelling of the throat, choking and dehydration
   d. Diarrhea, weight loss and electrolyte imbalance

2. All the serotonin (5-HT$_3$) receptor antagonists have what ending in their generic names?
   a. "tidine"
   b. "noid"
   c. "setron"
   d. "prazole"

3. Why are drugs that decrease prostaglandins like corticosteroids and NSAIDs harmful to the stomach?
   a. Decreased prostaglandins cause diarrhea, nausea, and vomiting.
   b. Prostaglandins are necessary for proper digestion.
   c. A decrease in prostaglandins will eventually cause bone loss and osteoporosis.
   d. Prostaglandins maintain good blood flow to the stomach, keeping tissues oxygenated.

4. All the histamine H$_2$ receptor antagonists have what ending in their generic names?
   a. "tidine"
   b. "noid"
   c. "setron"
   d. "prazole"

5. What issues are older adults more likely to experience as side effects of H$_2$ blockers compared with younger adults?
   a. Gastric ulcers
   b. Confusion and dizziness
   c. Nausea and vomiting
   d. Constipation

6. All the proton pump inhibitors have what ending in their generic names?
   a. "tidine"
   b. "noid"
   c. "setron"
   d. "prazole"

7. Why would a healthcare provider NOT provide an antidiarrheal to treat a patient's diarrhea?
   a. The patient does not have irritable bowel syndrome
   b. To help patient rid the body of an infection if the infection is causing the diarrhea
   c. To avoid side effects of antidiarrheals
   d. The patient is not experiencing dehydration

8. Which of the following is not an example of direct stimuli that can send messages to the vomiting center to cause nausea and vomiting?
   a. Cerebral cortex
   b. Vestibular apparatus
   c. Sensory organs
   d. Chemoreceptor trigger zone (CTZ)

9. Which class of antiemetic drugs are also called dopamine antagonists?
   a. Cannabinoids
   b. Substance P antagonists
   c. Serotonin (5-HT$_3$) receptor antagonists
   d. Phenothiazines

10. Antidepressants and St. John's wort should not be taken with:
    a. Cannabinoids
    b. Substance P antagonists
    c. Serotonin (5-HT$_3$) receptor antagonists
    d. Phenothiazines

11. When gastric distress causes destruction to the protective mucosal lining of the stomach, what can be produced if the lining is not repaired or gastric acid reduced?
    a. Duodenal and gastric ulcers
    b. Nausea and vomiting
    c. Constipation
    d. Diarrhea

12. What bacteria may also cause peptic ulcers?
    a. *Clostridium difficile*
    b. *E. coli*
    c. *H. pylori*
    d. *Salmonella*

13. Which is not a symptom of constipation?
    a. Fewer than three bowel movements per week
    b. Harder stools than normal
    c. Bowels still feeling full after a bowel movement
    d. Electrolyte imbalance

14. What is the best treatment for constipation?
    a. Cytoprotective drugs
    b. Healthy diet, adequate hydration, physical exercise
    c. Stool-softening drugs
    d. Osmotic drugs

15. When a patient has diarrhea due to a bacterial infection and cannot take antidiarrheals because it would slow down the body's ability to get rid of the organism, what is your role in supporting the patient?
    a. Diet and nutrition counseling
    b. Assisting in toileting
    c. Making sure that the patient has adequate hydration and skin care to prevent irritation to the anus
    d. Providing drugs to relieve pain and anxiety

85

Drugs Affecting the Hematologic System

MATCHING

Match the drugs listed in the left column with the drug categories on the right.

Drugs

1. _____ Reteplase

2. _____ Heparin

3. _____ Darbepoetin alfa

4. _____ Apixaban

5. _____ Aspirin

6. _____ Enoxaparin

7. _____ Clopidogrel

8. _____ Alteplase

9. _____ Rivaroxaban

10. _____ Warfarin

11. _____ Ferrous sulfate

Drug Categories

A. Platelet inhibitors
B. Direct thrombin inhibitors
C. Indirect thrombin inhibitors
D. Vitamin K antagonist
E. Fibrinolytics
F. Erythropoiesis-stimulating agents
G. Iron preparation

MATCHING

Match the term with the correct definition. (You may use the same answer more than once.)

Definitions

12. _____ Drugs that prevent platelets from clumping together (aggregating), which then interferes with blood clotting within arteries

13. _____ Drugs that use enzymes to dissolve the fibrin in a CLOT; Also known as thrombolytics or "clot busters"

14. _____ Drugs that convert plasminogen to the enzyme plasmin, which degrades or breaks down fibrin clots, fibrinogen, and other plasma proteins; used especially for *lysis* (dissolving) of thrombi

15. _____ An enzyme that acts on *fibrinogen* (a protein found in the blood plasma) to convert it to fibrin, which then helps clots to form.

16. _____ A protein found in the blood's plasma that is converted to fibrin to help form a blood clot

17. _____ Drugs that increase the time it takes for blood to clot, preventing new clots from forming

18. _____ A blockage in an artery by a blood clot or air bubble

19. _____ Anticoagulant drugs that prevent the formation of blood clots by interfering with the activity of the enzyme thrombin (factor II).

20. _____ Anticoagulant drugs that interfere with blood clotting by reducing the amount of vitamin K available to help the liver form clotting factors

21. _____ Anticoagulant drugs that reduce clot formation by increasing the protein antithrombin III

22. _____ Drugs that prevent clotting events in a patient who might be having reduced blood circulation to the heart before a *myocardial infarction* (heart attack)

23. _____ Drugs that are synthetic forms of the hormone *erythropoietin*, which stimulates the bone marrow to make more red blood cells at a faster rate

24. _____ A semisolid amount of coagulated (thickened) blood that blocks blood flow in a blood vessel; may also be referred to as a thrombus

25. _____ Products used to provide additional iron that is needed for producing hemoglobin and restoring body stores of iron

26. _____ A protein formed from fibrinogen that is a netlike substance in the blood with the function of trapping blood cells and platelets to form the matrix, or frame, of a clot during the clotting process

27. _____ A clot lying in a deep vein, usually in the legs

28. _____ Drugs that interfere with one or more steps in the blood-clotting process to either reduce or prevent new clots from forming, or prevent existing clots from getting larger

Terms

A. Anticoagulants
B. Clot
C. Deep vein thrombosis
D. Iron preparations
E. Direct thrombin inhibitors
F. Embolism
G. Erythropoiesis-stimulating agents (ESAs)
H. Fibrin
I. Fibrinogen
J. Fibrinolytic drugs
K. Indirect thrombin inhibitors
L. Platelet inhibitors
M. Thrombin
N. Vitamin K antagonists

29. Complete the table.

CATEGORY	SIDE EFFECTS	ADVERSE EFFECTS
Platelet inhibitors	_____ _____ _____ _____ _____ _____ _____	Excessive bleeding Allergic reactions to aspirin and NSAIDs Acute cardiovascular events can occur when these drugs are stopped abruptly Can result in a decrease in platelet counts (*thrombocytopenia*) and white blood cells counts (*neutropenia*)
Direct thrombin inhibitors	_____ _____ _____ _____ _____ _____ _____	Excessive bleeding Thrombocytopenia Early signs of overdose or internal bleeding include bleeding from the gums while brushing teeth, excessive bleeding or oozing from cuts, unexplained bruising, nosebleeds, and unusually heavy or unexpected menses in women
Indirect thrombin inhibitors	Can cause easy bleeding and bruising Pain, redness, warmth, irritation, or skin changes where the medicine was injected Foot itching Bluish-colored skin	_____ _____ _____ _____ _____ _____
Vitamin K antagonists	_____ _____ _____ _____ _____	Excessive bleeding or hemorrhage that can be seen with very heavy menstrual bleeding, frank blood or dark, tarry stools, or coffee-colored vomitus with excessive dosage Skin necrosis (death) Birth defects or death to the fetus
Iron preparations	Constipation, dark stool color, GI irritation, and nausea are the most common side effects Teeth can discolor with an oral preparation	_____ _____ _____ _____ _____ _____

CATEGORY	SIDE EFFECTS	ADVERSE EFFECTS
Fibrinolytic drugs	Bleeding Bleeding of the gums or injection or IV sites Low blood pressure (hypotension)	_____ _____ _____ _____ _____ _____ _____ _____
_____	Pain at the injection sites Generalized body aches and pain Skin rash Redness or warmth at the injection site	Higher risk for hypertension, blood clots, stroke, and myocardial infarction (heart attack) Increased tumor growth in some cancers Severe allergic reactions

MULTIPLE CHOICE

For each of the drug categories listed below, check all items that describe what should be taught to patients and families.

30. Platelet inhibitors

   a. _____ Take these drugs at least 2 hours before meals.

   b. _____ Look for symptoms of bleeding.

   c. _____ Avoid foods, supplements, and OTC drugs that can interfere with these drugs.

   d. _____ Do not stop taking these drugs for any reason.

31. Direct thrombin inhibitors

   a. _____ Look for signs of abnormal bleeding, including heavy menses.

   b. _____ Look for allergic reactions that include shortness of breath, facial swelling, rash, or hives.

   c. _____ Teach patients to take aspirin for aches and pains rather than other OTC drugs.

   d. _____ Pills should be removed from packaging and placed in plastic pill containers.

32. Indirect thrombin inhibitors

   a. _____ Look for signs of abnormal bleeding, including heavy menses.

   b. _____ Look for allergic reactions that include shortness of breath, facial swelling, rash, or hives.

   c. _____ Avoid aspirin or NSAIDs because of increased excessive bleeding risks.

   d. _____ Patients with latex allergies must find an alternative to these drugs.

33. Vitamin K antagonists

   a. _____ Patients MUST ensure they eat a sufficient amount of green, leafy vegetables to replace vitamin K deficiency.

   b. _____ Teach patients to keep all appointments for INR laboratory tests to determine proper dosage.

   c. _____ To avoid excessive bleeding, patients should not take aspirin or NSAIDs.

34. Fibrinolytics

   a. _____ Teach patients and family to administer this medication at home.

   b. _____ Ensure patients and family understand purpose, risks, and benefits.

   c. _____ Inform patients and family what symptoms to report after this drug has been administered.

35. Erythropoiesis-stimulating agents (ESAs)

  a. _____ The patient should check eight daily and report gains of 2 pounds within 24 hours or 4 pounds in a week due to possible water retention.

  b. _____ Assure patient that chest pains are normal side effects when taking this drug and there is no need to report this to the healthcare provider.

  c. _____ Patients must inform the healthcare provider if pregnant, breastfeeding, or planning to become pregnant.

36. Iron preparations

  a. _____ Take the oral tablet with a full glass of water.

  b. _____ Avoid aspirin while taking iron preparations.

  c. _____ Take any antihistamines as ordered during the treatment period.

  d. _____ Do not lie down for 10 minutes after taking ferrous sulfate

  e. _____ Prevent constipation by increasing water and fiber intake and taking a stool softener daily during treatment.

CASE STUDIES

Mrs. Davis, a 35-year-old female, is being treated with chemotherapy for cervical cancer. During a routine visit with her oncologist, she states that she has felt extreme weakness and fatigue during the past week. She said she felt like she did a few months ago when she had anemia and was given a blood transfusion. After examining her, the oncologist ordered a CBC. The results from the lab show her RBC count, hemoglobin, and hematocrit are all exceptionally low. She is diagnosed with anemia and will be treated with erythropoiesis-stimulating agents (ESAs) instead of a blood transfusion to avoid complications of transfusions such as fluid overload.

1. Mrs. Davis asks about the risks or adverse side effects involved with ESAs. What will you explain to her? (Check all that apply.)
   1. Mrs. Davis's blood can become thicker as the RBC production increases, which can cause blood clots, hypertension, stroke, and MI (heart attack)
   2. Shortness of breath, wheezing, chest tightness, facial swelling, skin rash, or hives can occur.
   3. ESA can cause water retention and increase blood pressure.
   4. ESA can increase the growth of cancer cells in advanced cancers.
   5. There are risks for severe allergic reactions to the ESA treatment.
   6. If unsuccessful, Mrs. Davis may still require a transfusion.
   7. Hemorrhage is the most critical adverse reaction.
   8. ESAs can often be responsible for severe bleeding.

2. Mrs. Davis also asked about the usual side effects that may occur. What expected side effects can you tell her about? (Select all that apply.)
   1. Pain at the injection site is the most common side effect of ESAs.
   2. Bleeding of the gums or injection or IV sites can occur.
   3. Low blood pressure can occur.
   4. Generalized body aches and pain, skin rash, redness, or warmth at the injection site can occur.
   5. Intense nausea occurs 2 to 3 hours after the injection.
   6. High blood pressure can occur.

Reggie Jones is a 35-year-old man who lives alone and works in an IT department. He works long hours and often forgets to eat. As a result, he has developed an iron deficiency and is very weak and sleepy. His healthcare provider recommends he pay more attention to his diet and take ferrous sulfate 325 mg tablets three times daily.

3. What signs and symptoms will you assess for in Reggie Jones? (Select all that apply.)
   1. Allergic reactions
   2. Signs of anaphylaxis
   3. Excessive WBCs
   4. Skin and mucous membrane color
   5. Hair loss
   6. His CBC

PRACTICE QUIZ

1. Why is it important for blood to flow freely through blood vessels?
   a. It distributes waste products in the bloodstream to organs such as kidneys.
   b. It provides cells with oxygen and nutrients.
   c. It protects cells from excesses of enzymes.
   d. It prevents clotting of blood.

2. What is the most common reason for blood beginning to clot?
   a. Deficiency of the thrombin enzyme
   b. Excessive vitamin K within the bloodstream
   c. Damage to the blood vessels or tissues
   d. Lack of sufficient red blood cells

3. If the arteries become plugged with thrombi (clots of fibrin, platelets, and cholesterol), what can happen to the body's tissues?
   a. Oxygen is prohibited from reaching the tissues, which may result in death.
   b. Emboli can break off and cause bleeding in other parts of the body.
   c. Clots can damage legs or ankles and cause permanent neuropathy.
   d. Glucose is prohibited from reaching the muscles, which may cause weakness.

91

4. How do anticoagulants interfere in the clotting process?
   a. Thin the blood
   b. Reduce or prevent new clots from forming
   c. Dissolve existing clots
   d. Prevent clots from breaking off as emboli

5. How do fibrinolytic drugs interfere in the clotting process?
   a. Prevent plasminogen from converting to plasmin
   b. Provide plasma proteins to protect the tissue
   c. Emergency drug carried by patient to use when they determine clot is forming
   d. Dissolve and break down existing blood clots

6. How does platelet aggregation protect the body when it is injured?
   a. Platelet aggregation prevents clots in the cardiovascular system.
   b. Platelet aggregation keeps the blood thin so that clots are unable to be formed when there are injuries.
   c. Platelets aggregate and seal the entry to the vascular system to prevent blood from accessing the body tissues.
   d. Platelets aggregate and inhibit clots from breaking off and moving to other parts of the body.

7. What is a common sign of excessive bleeding that patients need to notice?
   a. Frequent, heavy nosebleeds
   b. Bleeding from the gums when brushing teeth
   c. Bleeding around the cuticles when washing hands or feet
   d. Unusually reddened eyes

8. Which of the following can increase bleeding or decrease the effectiveness of an anticoagulant drug?
   a. Red meat
   b. Diet cola
   c. St. John's wort
   d. Acetaminophen

9. Which of the following drug types are frequently given for atrial fibrillation?
   a. Direct thrombin inhibitors
   b. Indirect thrombin inhibitors
   c. Vitamin K antagonist
   d. Fibrinolytics

10. What is low-molecular-weight especially used to prevent?
    a. Venous thromboembolism
    b. Pulmonary embolism
    c. Cardiac arrest
    d. Dysrhythmia

11. What is the most commonly used blood test for determining the therapeutic range for heparin?
    a. Activated partial thromboplastin time
    b. Prothrombin time
    c. International normalized ratio
    d. PT/INR

12. Within how many hours after the onset of a stroke must fibrinolytics be started to dissolve the blood clot blocking the artery?
    a. Within 12 hours
    b. Within 3 hours
    c. Within 6 hours
    d. Within 4–8 hours

13. What happens when red blood cell (RBC) counts fall due to anemia?
    a. The liver secretes the hormone thrombopoietin, which travels to the bone marrow.
    b. Patients must be treated with supplements to increase RBC production and receive further treatment with ESAs.
    c. The kidneys secrete the hormone erythropoietin, which stimulates production of RBCs.
    d. Patients require a bone marrow transplant and injections of ESAs.

14. Which of the following drug types can help reduce the need for transfusions?
    a. Indirect thrombin inhibitors
    b. Vitamin K antagonist
    c. Fibrinolytics
    d. Erythropoiesis-stimulating agents

15. What should patients taking anticoagulants do prior to dental surgical procedures?
    a. Discontinue the drug prior to surgery to avoid bleeding issues
    b. Ensure all procedures are done within a fully equipped surgical facility
    c. Discontinue the drug after the surgery for at least 72 hours
    d. Work with healthcare provider to provide another drug less likely to cause bleeding issues

16. Which one of the following is NOT a reason for administering parenteral iron rather than giving the patient oral iron supplements?
    a. The patient cannot tolerate oral iron supplements.
    b. The healthcare provider want to prevent cardiac arrest.
    c. Oral supplements are not effective for the patient.
    d. The patient requires an immediate increase of iron stores.

16 Drugs for Immunization and Immunomodulation

TYPES OF IMMUNITY

Indicate for each description in the left column what type of immunity is applicable.

Descriptions

1. _____ A 30-year-old man is bitten by a rabid raccoon. He had not been previously vaccinated for rabies. He receives a series of injections that contain antibodies created by other individuals who had rabies. Once the shots are discontinued, his body destroys the antibodies that were not created in his body.

2. _____ A woman and her infant are exposed to a disease for which the woman has developed antibodies within her body. She is currently breast-feeding the infant, and the infant resists the disease as well.

3. _____ A patient who previously had strep throat is exposed again. Her body already has antibodies prepared to destroy the bacteria and the effects of the disease are much less severe. She develops more antibodies and when she is exposed again, the bacteria are destroyed before causing any disease.

4. _____ A 60-year-old man receives a pneumonia vaccine, which contains a few microorganisms of the disease, and his body creates protective antibodies to the pneumococcal bacteria without actually having been exposed to the disease. He will likely need booster shots to ensure his antibodies remain active.

5. _____ A patient is exposed to the *Streptococcus pyogenes* bacteria (strep throat) and immediately, her body begins developing antibodies to fight off the cells that do not contain her genetic code.

Types of Immunity

A. Innate immunity
B. Natural acquired active immunity
C. Natural acquired passive immunity
D. Artificial acquired active immunity
E. Artificial acquired passive immunity

NURSING RESPONSIBILITY FOR ADMINISTERING VACCINATIONS

6. Number each of the items listed below in the order you would perform the action.

_____ Unpack and store vials in designated area within the refrigerator, separate from other drugs

_____ Observe the patient for any immediate reactions

_____ Inject the vaccine using recommended technique and site

_____ Check the expiration date on the vaccine vial

_____ Draw up the appropriate dose

_____ Document all required information

_____ Tell the patient what side effects could be expected

_____ Ask the patient if he ever had a reaction to the vaccine or components

VACCINATION SCHEDULES

7. For each age shown on the timeline, write above or below the timeline which of the vaccination(s) and/or booster(s) is recommended.
   a. DTaP
   b. DTaP booster
   c. Tdap
   d. Tdap booster
   e. Pneumonia
   f. Influenza
   g. Shingles

| 2 mos | 4 mos | 6 mos | 15–18 mos | 4–6 yrs | 11–12 yrs | 19 yrs | 19, 29, 39 yrs, etc. | 65 yrs |

8. For each of the diseases listed below, indicate whether a vaccine should be given in (a) childhood, (b) adulthood, (c) based on vocation/travel.

   _____ Malaria

   _____ HPV

   _____ Typhoid

   _____ Hepatitis A and B

   _____ Measles, mumps, rubella (MMR)

   _____ Polio

   _____ Pertussis

   _____ Rabies

9. Select which of the following vaccines can be given to women <u>during</u> pregnancy.

   _____ Measles, mumps, rubella (MMR)

   _____ Seasonal influenza

   _____ Tdap

   _____ Chicken pox

   _____ Polio

IDENTIFYING SELECTIVE IMMUNOSUPPRESSANT DRUGS

Identify for each drug listed in the left column the correct drug category listed in the right column.

Drugs

10. _____ Mycophenolate

11. _____ Cyclosporine

12. _____ Sirolimus

13. _____ Azathioprine

14. _____ Tacrolimus

15. _____ Everolimus

Drug Categories

A. Antiproliferative drugs
B. Calcineurin drugs

94

FILL IN THE BLANK

Using the list of drugs from the previous exercise above, fill in the name of the drug to match the descriptions.

16. _____ selectively suppresses T- and B-lymphocytes activity by inhibiting an enzyme needed for lymphocyte reproduction and prevents T-cell activation.

17. _____ inhibits T-cell activation and reproduction, blocking the mTOR signal pathways that promote completion of cell division for T cells. Fewer T cells lead to less tumor necrosis factor and other substances that can attack normal tissues and transplanted organs.

18. _____ inhibits the mTOR pathway so lymphocyte cell division and growth are reduced. It is more specific against immune system cells that attack normal self-cells and transplanted organs than general antiproliferative drugs.

19. _____ and _____ are calcineurin inhibitors and work by forming a complex around the normal calcineurin present inside T lymphocytes, preventing the calcineurin from activating those cells. With less ability to be activated, the T cells are not able to attack and damage transplanted tissues and organs.

TRUE OR FALSE

Indicate whether each of the following statements are true or false.

20. _____ Selective immunosuppressants are safe for use, even if a patient has a systemic infection.

21. _____ Tacrolimus can cause diabetes mellitus.

22. _____ Sirolimus is the only selective immunosuppressant that increases blood cholesterol levels.

23. _____ Calcineurin inhibitors increase blood cholesterol and blood glucose levels.

24. _____ Patients taking selective immunosuppressants are at an increased risk for cancer.

25. _____ Phlebitis and thrombosis can be adverse effects when patients are taking calcineurin inhibitors orally.

26. _____ Liver failure can occur with all selective immunosuppressants.

27. _____ Antiproliferatives are the only selective immunosuppressants that can cause imbalances of potassium, phosphorus, and magnesium.

28. _____ Patients taking selective immunosuppressants should ensure they are vaccinated with all possible options to prevent infections.

SHORT ANSWER

Answer the questions below, indicating how you would teach patients and their families about the following concerns.

29. What are at least five signs that may be indicative of a potential infection and should be monitored daily by patients or their families?

_____

_____

30. What are at least three signs that may be indicative of potential liver toxicity and should be monitored daily by patients or their families?

_____

_____

31. Name two substances the patient should avoid to prevent liver damage when taking immunosuppressant drugs.

_____

_____

32. Why is it important for the patient to take the drugs exactly as prescribed?

_____

_____

33. Describe how to teach the patient to effectively administer the oral suspensions of sirolimus or cyclosporine.

_____

_____

_____

34. If taking sirolimus as well as cyclosporine, when should the drugs be administered to ensure the best effect?

_____

_____

35. Why should sirolimus or tacrolimus not be taken with grapefruit juice?

_____

_____

CASE STUDIES

Mrs. Agnes Jones, a 72-year-old female patient, is refusing her annual influenza vaccination because she had read on the Internet that she could possibly have serious reactions to the vaccination. Mrs. Jones feels getting the flu might be preferable to the adverse side effects she had read about. She had also read that it was not necessary to have the vaccination every year because she had the flu last year and thought she would still have immunity.

1. What is the most appropriate response by the nurse to Mrs. Jones regarding the adverse side effects? (Choose the most appropriate response.)
   1. "You should discuss your decision to refuse the vaccination with your healthcare provider."
   2. "There is some risk for adverse side effects such as a fever over 103°F (39.4°C), anaphylactic shock, seizures, and neuropathy. However, the risk for these rare complications outweighs the risk for the serious problems that disease can cause for both you and all others who come in contact with you."
   3. "Expected side effects and any adverse reactions associated with each of them can be found on the CDC website."
   4. "Vaccines are carefully monitored for safety."

2. What should the nurse explain to Mrs. Jones about yearly influenza vaccinations? (Choose all that apply.)
   1. "If you got sick with one specific strain last year, you would develop active immunity to it. However, each year, different strains may come to your community."
   2. "We don't allow patients in this clinic who are not vaccinated against influenza."
   3. "It is recommended for adults and children to receive a seasonal influenza vaccination every year."
   4. "You should think of protecting all the other persons who may not have as strong an immune system as you do."
   5. "You should be assessed for antibodies by having a blood titer performed before deciding about taking the influenza vaccination."
   6. "You really shouldn't believe what you read on the Internet. Most of the information on there isn't true."
   7. "The vaccination contains antigens for the three or four viruses that are predicted by the CDC to be the most common ones prevalent this year. Receiving the vaccination helps you develop active immunity only to these three or four influenza strains, which then protects you against those strains for a long time. However, this year, the most commonly predicted strains may not be the ones you were vaccinated against last year. So if you skip this year's vaccination, you may not have any immunity to the different strains of influenza."
   8. "An influenza vaccination will also help prevent colds and pneumonia."

Sarah Moore is a 35-year-old woman with two young children. She recently had a kidney transplant, which was donated by her brother. One of the drugs prescribed by her healthcare provider is CellCept. She is nervous about the drug and concerned about what she can expect. As a mother, she is worried about taking care of her children. This increases her anxiousness. You want to prepare her so she will be able to identify any problems.

3. What other warnings should Sarah have before she begins the drug? (Select all that apply.)
   1. Look for signs of bleeding.
   2. Avoid taking aspirin.
   3. Exercise should be limited.
   4. Schedule a BUN and creatinine level test on a regular basis.
   5. Look for signs of renal failure such as a decrease in urine output.
   6. Report nausea and vomiting if accompanied by fever and diarrhea.
   7. Avoid taking CellCept with grapefruit juice.
   8. You do not need to take vaccinations such as yearly influenza vaccines.

4. When Sarah comes in for the next visit, she informs you that she and her husband are trying to get pregnant. What is your response?
   1. She must stop taking CellCept for at least 6 weeks before trying to get pregnant.
   2. Getting pregnant is no longer a possibility.
   3. CellCept unfortunately causes infertility.
   4. She must stop taking CellCept for a year before trying to get pregnant.

PRACTICE QUIZ

1. Which of the following best describes innate immunity?
   a. It occurs when all vaccinations have been taken as scheduled as children and the individual is protected by antibodies.
   b. It occurs when the body recognizes foreign cells invading the body and acts by developing antibodies.
   c. It occurs when the body is invaded by common diseases and family members or close acquaintances are not infected.
   d. It occurs when adult vaccinations are taken on a regular basis.

2. Which of the following best describes acquired immunity?
   a. It occurs when the body is exposed to microorganisms after already having built antigens to destroy it.
   b. It occurs from vaccinations.
   c. It occurs when newborns acquire it from the mother in vitro.
   d. It occurs when a current infection within the body prevents other infections from taking hold.

3. Immunity acquired through vaccinations is referred to as which of the following types?
   a. Natural acquired active immunity
   b. Natural acquired passive immunity
   c. Artificial acquired active immunity
   d. Artificial acquired passive immunity

4. Why do vaccinations target B cells to stimulate antibody production?
   a. B cells are located in the lymphatic system.
   b. B cells are capable of helping the body develop natural immunity.
   c. B cells are the most prolific cells found in the body.
   d. B cells are the only WBC that can form antibodies in response to the vaccine.

5. What is the difference between vaccination and immunization?
   a. Vaccinations refer to shots with live cultures; immunizations refer to shots containing antibodies.
   b. Vaccinations are generally for children and immunizations refer to adults.
   c. Vaccinations are the actual shots and immunization is what occurs within the body.
   d. Vaccinations and immunizations are used interchangeably.

6. What types of vaccines are composed of chemically modified microorganisms?
   a. Inactivated vaccines
   b. Attenuated vaccines
   c. Toxoid vaccines
   d. Biosynthetic vaccines

7. What types of vaccines are composed of microorganisms that have been killed?
   a. Inactivated vaccines
   b. Attenuated vaccines
   c. Toxoid vaccines
   d. Biosynthetic vaccines

8. What types of vaccines are composed of genetically engineered microorganisms?
   a. Inactivated vaccines
   b. Attenuated vaccines
   c. Toxoid vaccines
   d. Biosynthetic vaccines

9. What types of vaccines are composed of weakened but live organisms?
   a. Inactivated vaccines
   b. Attenuated vaccines
   c. Toxoid vaccines
   d. Biosynthetic vaccines

10. What occurs in the body when an individual develops an autoimmune disorder?
    a. The body keeps developing antibodies after the foreign microorganism has been destroyed and the antibodies enter the bloodstream.
    b. Autoimmune disorders occur after receiving a blood transfusion and foreign substances attack the organs.
    c. The immune system views normal body tissue as foreign and attacks it.
    d. The immune system has been suppressed due to chemical substances and prevents appropriate response when a foreign substance invades the body.

11. Why are selective immunosuppressant drugs preferred to nonselective immunosuppressant drugs for patients with autoimmune diseases?
    a. Select immunosuppressant drugs target the affected area, reducing infection risk.
    b. Nonselective immunosuppressant drugs are not effective for most autoimmune diseases.
    c. Select immunosuppressant drugs are created from the patients' antibodies, which helps reduce risks of immune dysfunction.
    d. Nonselective immunosuppressant drugs must be given at significantly higher dosages.

12. In addition to autoimmune diseases such as rheumatoid arthritis, what other condition requires immunosuppressant drugs?
    a. Osteoarthritis
    b. Joint replacements
    c. Organ transplants
    d. Influenza

13. Which types of drugs can cause phlebitis and/or thrombosis when given intravenously?
    a. Calcineurin inhibitors
    b. Antiproliferatives
    c. Toxoids
    d. Tdap

14. How do antirejection drugs work to protect a patient who has received an organ transplant?
    a. They create antibodies that ensure diseases do not impact the transplanted organ.
    b. They modify toxoids chemically so they are no longer toxic.
    c. They suppress the cells and factors of the immune system.
    d. They prevent rejection by generating microorganisms that project the transplanted organ.

15. What is the purpose in performing an antibody titer on a patient?
    a. To detect and measure the amount of a specific antibody in the person's blood to determine the person's immunity
    b. To identify the types of antibodies already present in a person's blood to determine which vaccines are actually needed
    c. To test a patient with autoimmune disease to determine whether a vaccine will cause an adverse reaction
    d. To determine whether an organism that can damage tissue is in the person's system

17 Drugs for Osteoporosis and Hormonal Problems

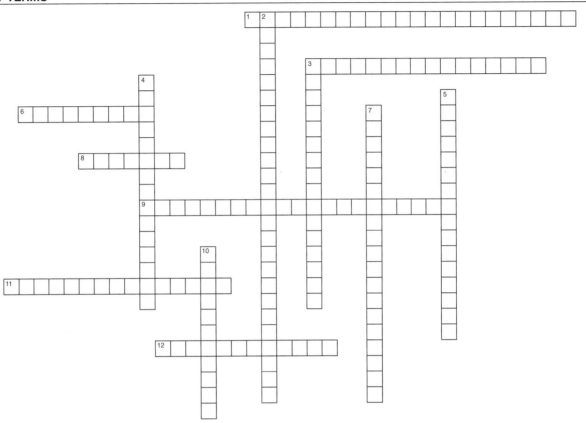

ACROSS

1. Drugs that mimic effects of thyroid hormones T3 and T4, helping to regulate metabolism
3. Thyroid-suppressing drugs that work directly in the thyroid gland to stop production of new hormones by preventing an enzyme from connects iodine (iodide) with tyrosine to make active thyroid hormones
6. Synthetic or natural hormones that help to develop and maintain the male sex organs at puberty and develop secondary sex characteristics in men (facial hair, deep voice, body hair, body fat distribution, and muscle development).
8. A protein secreted by an endocrine gland that changes the action of another gland or tissue, known as its target tissue
9. The use of hormones to suppress ovulation for the intentional prevention of pregnancy
11. Drugs similar to natural cortisol, a hormone secreted by the adrenal cortex that is essential for life
12. The gradual loss of bone density and strength, which leads to spinal shortening and increased risk for bone fractures

DOWN

2. Temporary or permanent therapy with drugs that perform the function of natural endocrine hormones
3. Synthetic drugs with the same use and actions as androgens
4. Calcium-modifying drugs that both prevent bones from losing calcium and increase bone density by moving blood calcium into the bone, binding to calcium in the bone, and preventing osteoclasts from destroying bone cells and reabsorbing calcium
5. Drugs for osteoporosis that activate (agonize) estrogen receptors in the bone to promote calcium retention in the bone
7. Drugs for osteoporosis that block estrogen receptors in breast and uterine tissue
10. A hormone secreted by the adrenal cortex that regulates sodium and water balance

99

THE ENDOCRINE SYSTEM

Fill in the blanks to the following questions regarding endocrine glands and hormone replacement therapy (HRT).

1. Why are the endocrine glands known as "ductless" glands?

   _____

   _____

2. How do the hormones produced by the endocrine glands reach their target tissue?

   _____

   _____

3. Hormone replacement therapy (HRT) is used when endocrine glands cannot produce the adequate amount of hormone. Name the common uses of HRT.

   a. _____

   b. _____

   c. _____

   d. _____

   e. _____

4. Depending on how important the function of the hormone is to a patient's health and well-being, HRT can be used for a short time or permanently. Give an example of each circumstance.

   a. Short-term _____

   b. Permanently _____

5. Hormones are regulated by a _____ loop. Give an example of an undesirable consequence when the regulation process has a defect in the patients' blood glucose.

   a. _____.

DRUGS FOR THYROID PROBLEMS

Fill in the blanks for the following questions regarding drugs for thyroid problems.

6. Name the two thyroid hormones necessary for life.

   _____

7. Name the body actions that the thyroid hormones control.

   a. _____

   b. _____

   c. _____

   d. _____

8. _____ is a condition when there is little or no production of the thyroid hormones.

9. _____ are drugs that mimic the effect of the thyroid hormones T3 and T4, helping to regulate metabolism.

10. Side effects of this class of drugs are:

_____

_____

_____

_____

11. List the possible adverse reactions that may occur with thyroid hormone agonists.

a. _____

_____

b. _____

_____

12. _____ is a condition in which the thyroid gland secretes excessive amounts of thyroid hormones (T3 and T4). The most common cause is _____.

13. Severe hyperthyroidism that causes life-threatening hypertension, heart failure, and seizures is called thyroid _____ or thyroid _____. Often, a _____ is the first indication of the problem. This condition is an emergency and can lead to death if the thyroid hormone levels are not decreased immediately.

14. _____ work directly in the thyroid gland to stop production of the hormones.

15. The names of these drugs are _____ and _____, which belong to the thionamide class of drugs.

16. Side effects of antithyroid drugs can include:

_____

_____

_____

_____

17. List the possible adverse effects of antithyroid drugs.

a. _____

b. _____

c. _____

d. _____

101

18. Indicate which statements are important to teach patients and families about thyroid hormone agonists (**T**) and which are important for antithyroid drugs (**A**). Some of the statements will be true for both classes of drugs.

_____ You must take the drug daily to maintain normal body function and not skip doses.

_____ Take the missed dose as soon as you remember it. However, if it is almost time for the next dose, skip the missed dose and continue your regular dosing schedule. Do not take a double dose to make up for a missed one.

_____ Take the drug 2 to 3 hours before a meal or taking a fiber supplement, or at least 3 hours after a meal or taking the supplement because food and fiber greatly decrease absorption of the drug.

_____ Take only the dose that is prescribed for you because increasing the drug too quickly can lead to adverse effects such as a heart attack or seizures.

_____ Keep all follow-up appointments and appointments for blood-clotting tests because these drugs increase the effectiveness of warfarin.

_____ If you are ill and cannot take the drug orally, contact your healthcare provider to get an injection dose of the drug.

_____ Go to the emergency department immediately if you start to have chest pain.

_____ Even if you do not notice a reduction of your symptoms in the first 1 to 2 weeks, do not increase the dosage on your own. These drugs take several weeks to be effective.

_____ Do not stop the drug suddenly or change the dose (up or down) without contacting your healthcare provider to prevent underdosing or overdosing.

_____ Check your pulse each morning before taking the drug and again each evening before going to bed. If the pulse rate becomes 20 beats higher than the normal rate for 1 week or if it becomes consistently irregular, notify your healthcare provider.

_____ Check the color of the roof of your mouth and the whites of your eyes daily for a yellow tinge that may indicate a liver problem. If this appears, notify your healthcare provider as soon as possible.

_____ Avoid situations that can lead to bleeding and other drugs that can make bleeding worse.

_____ Avoid crowds and people who are ill because these drugs can reduce your immunity and resistance to infection.

DRUGS FOR ADRENAL GLAND PROBLEMS

Fill in the blanks for the following statements regarding the adrenal glands.

19. What are the corticosteroid hormones produced by the cortex of the adrenal gland?

_____

20. _____ controls sodium and water balance. Because it regulates sodium, it is also known as a

_____.

21. _____ helps maintain critical blood glucose levels, the stress response, excitability of cardiac muscle, immunity, and blood sodium levels.

22. Cortisol was first discovered to affect blood glucose levels; it is also known as a _____.

23. _____ is a disorder in which the adrenal gland produces little or no cortisol and aldosterone.

24. When adrenal gland _____ occurs, only one hormone is oversecreted. Excessive secretion of cortisol is

known as _____ or _____. Excessive secretion of aldosterone is _____.

25. _____ is the most common treatment for adrenal gland hyperfunction. Drug therapy can also be used.

MATCHING

Match the correct term to the descriptions regarding adrenal gland problems and the actions, side effects, and adverse reactions of the drugs used to treat those problems. You may use the terms more than once and some descriptions may match more than one term.

Descriptions

26. _____ Conditions that cause it include autoimmune disease attacking and destroying the adrenal glands, adrenalectomy, abdominal radiation therapy, and reduced function of the anterior pituitary gland. Major problems are *hypoglycemia*, salt wasting, hypotension, weakness, and high blood potassium levels

27. _____ The most common cause of this condition is an adrenal gland tumor. Sometimes a problem in the pituitary gland is responsible.

28. _____ Both of these can cause the adverse effect of adrenal insufficiency.

29. _____ Used for hormone replacement therapy, but their most common use is as powerful antiinflammatory drugs.

30. _____ A steroid production inhibitor that works by directly preventing adrenal gland production of cortisol and other adrenal cortex hormones

31. _____ Drugs that act just like natural cortisol. Because they have some effect on sodium balance, most patients with adrenal gland hypofunction only need hormone replacement therapy with these.

32. _____ This drug works by blocking corticosteroid receptors. Although this does not reduce cortisol levels, it does inhibit cortisol responses in different tissues.

33. _____ A synthetic drug that acts like natural aldosterone. With the use of this drug, more sodium is retained to prevent excessive sodium wasting, and more potassium is excreted to prevent dangerously high blood potassium levels. So it helps prevent hyponatremia, hyperkalemia, and hypotension.

34. _____ Drug therapy for this condition focuses on reducing potassium levels and relies on spironolactone (Aldactone, Spironol, Novo-Spiroton), a potassium-sparing diuretic.

35. _____ Side effects include hypertension, edema formation, low blood potassium levels, and high blood sodium levels. The cause of these problems is the drug's action on fluid and electrolyte balance.

36. _____ Allergic reaction can occur. Emergency help is needed for hives; difficult breathing; and swelling of the face, lips, tongue, or throat. Used to induce abortions and can cause pregnancy loss.

37. _____ Congestive heart failure (CHF) is a serious adverse effect of this drug. It requires that the drug dose be either reduced or stopped.

38. _____ Cause nausea, vomiting, skin rashes, and dizziness. This drug can also cause bloody urine (hematuria).

39. _____ Cause nausea, vomiting, skin rashes, and dizziness. This drug can also cause menstrual irregularities.

Terms

A. Glucocorticoids, especially prednisone
B. Fludrocortisone (Florinef)
C. Mitotane (Lysodren)
D. Mifepristone (Korlym)
E. Adrenal gland hypofunction
F. Adrenal gland hyperfunction (hypercortisolism, Cushing's disease, hyperaldosteronism)

TEACHING PATIENTS AND FAMILIES ABOUT DRUGS FOR ADRENAL PROBLEMS

Fill in the blank for each of the topics below that describe important information the patient and their families should be aware of when taking drugs for adrenal problems.

40. Take _____ at the same time daily with food to prevent _____ problems.

41. Weigh yourself daily and keep a record because adrenal gland hypofunction drugs can cause fluid retention with

    _____ _____.

42. Report a weight gain of _____ lb. in a day or _____ lb. in a week to the healthcare provider immediately when taking adrenal gland hypofunction drugs.

43. Keep all appointments for laboratory blood work because adrenal gland hyperfunction drugs alter blood levels of

    _____ and _____.

44. When taking drugs for adrenal gland hyperfunction, report symptoms of adrenal insufficiency to your healthcare provider immediately. These include:

    _____

    _____

45. Take adrenal gland hyperfunction drugs with food because they all can cause _____, _____, and other gastrointestinal upsets.

46. If you are a sexually active woman in your childbearing years, use two reliable forms of _____ while

    taking _____ because this drug can cause a pregnancy loss.

DRUGS FOR SEX HORMONE REPLACEMENT AND CONTRACEPTION

Fill in the blank for the topics below regarding the uses and actions of sex hormone replacement and contraception.

47. _____ hormone replacement therapy (HRT) during the _____ period is the replacement

    of naturally secreted _____ and _____ with hormones given in the form of a drug.

48. Oral contraceptives provide enough _____ to interfere with feedback and decrease the body's natural

    production of estrogen and progesterone. As a result, _____ stops and the _____ mucus thickens, making fertilization difficult.

49. _____ are steroid hormones synthesized from _____, and they work to stimulate or control the development and maintenance of male characteristics.

50. Giving a woman low doses of _____ increases blood estrogen levels. This action reduces

    _____.

51. The most effective oral contraceptives contain two synthetic hormones, a _____ and _____, a synthetic progesterone. When taken consistently, this hormone combination keeps the blood levels of estrogen and

    progesterone high, signaling the _____ that further secretion of these hormones is not needed.

52. Androgens are primarily used in the treatment of hypogonadism, hypopituitarism, *eunuchism* (absence of testes or undeveloped gonads in a male), *cryptorchidism* (undescended testes), *oligospermia* (lack of sperm in the semen), and

    general androgen deficiency in males. The most commonly used androgen is _____.

53. _____ are oral contraceptives that contain only progestin rather than a combination of estrogen and progestin.

    They increase blood levels of _____, turning off the hormone pathway with positive feedback, which prevents

    _____. They are not as effective as combination oral contraceptives and most must be taken daily.

MATCHING

Match the name of the drug with the description of its side effects and adverse reactions. You may use the drugs more than once. Some descriptions may match more than one drug.

Descriptions

54. _____ Side effects include breast tenderness, breakthrough bleeding, fluid retention, weight gain, and acne.

55. _____ Adverse reactions may include heart attack, increased risk of blood clotting, excessive bleeding, risk of hormone-sensitive cancers, liver impairment, gallstones, and pancreatitis.

56. _____ Adverse reactions with long-term, high-dose therapy could be liver tumor, liver cancer and hepatitis. Other possible adverse effects could include jaundice, a decreased sperm count, *gynecomastia*, impotence, and urinary retention

57. _____ Adverse reactions may include blood clot formation, hypertension, liver toxicity, growth of hormone-sensitive cancers, increase of serum potassium level and interaction with other drugs that increase potassium levels.

58. _____ Side effects include edema caused by sodium retention, acne, *hirsutism*, male pattern baldness, mouth irritation, diarrhea, nausea, and vomiting.

Drugs

A. Perimenopausal HRT drugs
B. Oral contraceptives
C. Androgens

TEACHING PATIENTS AND FAMILIES ABOUT SEX HORMONE REPLACEMENT AND CONTRACEPTION DRUGS

Fill in the blank for each topic below regarding what is important to teach patients and families about sex hormone replacement and contraception drugs

59. Quit or reduce _____ during the time you take perimenopausal HRT and oral contraceptive drugs to reduce your risk for blood clots, heart attacks, and strokes.

60. Check the color of the roof of your mouth and the whites of your eyes weekly for the presence of a _____ tinge because perimenopausal HRT and oral contraceptive drugs can impair the _____. If you see this yellowing, report it to your healthcare provider as soon as possible.

61. Use an additional method of _____ during the first cycle because oral contraceptives require a full cycle before they are effective.

62. Take the oral contraceptive with _____ once daily at the same time each day for best effect and to remember to take it. Oral contraceptives are only _____ if taken as _____.

63. Make sure your healthcare provider is aware of other prescribed drugs or over-the-counter drugs you are taking in order to avoid _____.

64. Do not increase the dose of _____ without consulting your healthcare provider if you do not see the expected effects within the first _____ months because response to the drug may take several months.

65. When taking androgen steroids, report any new or troublesome symptoms that may develop, including:

_____

_____

_____

66. If you are taking androgen steroids _____ or _____, for best absorption, do not eat, drink, smoke, or chew tobacco until the drug is dissolved.

67. If you are using a _____ form of the drug, do not let women or children come into contact with the areas where you have applied it to prevent them from absorbing the drug.

105

DRUGS FOR OSTEOPOROSIS

Match the name of the drug with the correct description of the actions, uses, side effects, and adverse reactions. You may use the names of the drugs more than once.

Descriptions

68. _____ Calcium-modifying drugs that prevent bones from losing calcium and increase by moving blood calcium into the bone, binding to calcium in the bone, and preventing osteoclasts from destroying bone cells and resorbing calcium. They also prevent certain white blood cells from damaging or destroying bone.

69. _____ Common side effects of these drugs are muscle spasms, nausea, and indigestion. Some people have hot flashes, sodium retention, and edema formation.

70. _____ This drug can cause allergic reactions and possible anaphylaxis. The risk increases with repeated dosage of the drug. Jaw osteonecrosis also can occur.

71. _____ Common side effects are headache, esophageal reflux, and nausea.

72. _____ Drugs that activate estrogen receptors in the bone to promote calcium retention in the bone and block estrogen receptors in breast tissue and uterine tissue. These opposing responses increase bone density and prevent excessive growth of breast tissue that can lead to cancer and overgrowth of uterine endometrial tissues that can lead to excessive uterine bleeding.

73. _____ Skin rashes and muscle and joint pain are the most common side effects.

74. _____ A possible adverse effect is the increased risk for thrombotic events, which include deep vein thrombosis, stroke, myocardial infarction, and pulmonary embolism.

75. _____ Antibodies directed against immature osteoclasts. Binding of the antibodies to these cells prevents them from maturing and reducing bone density.

76. _____ Jawbone necrosis (*osteonecrosis*) can develop with tooth extraction or other invasive dental procedures in which the jawbone is damaged. This adverse reaction is more common in patients taking higher doses or the intravenous form of the drug.

77. _____ Additional uses are the prevention of skeletal fractures in patients with bone metastases and multiple myeloma, Paget's disease, and the treatment of cancer-induced hypercalcemia.

78. _____ These drugs stimulate osteoclast activity, which results in the formation of new bone growth. They are especially useful for patients who have a high risk for fractures and in whom other treatments have failed.

Drugs

A. Bisphosphonates
B. Estrogen agonists/ antagonists
C. Osteoclast monoclonal antibodies
D. Sclerostin inhibitors

TEACHING PATIENTS AND FAMILIES ABOUT DRUGS FOR OSTEOPOROSIS

Fill in the blank for each topic below regarding what is important to teach patients and families about drugs for osteoporosis.

79. Take bisphosphonates early in the morning, right after breakfast, and _____.

80. Remain in the upright position (sitting, standing, or walking) for at least _____ after taking these drugs to prevent esophageal irritation and reflux.

81. Do not _____ while taking estrogen agonists/antagonists to prevent forming dangerous blood clots that could cause a stroke or heart attack.

106

82. Avoid excessive _____ and _____ intake to prevent _____.

83. If you start having _____ or just don't feel right when you are receiving osteo-clast monoclonal antibodies, call for help immediately.

84. Be sure to inform your dentist or oral surgeon that you are taking a _____ or receiving _____ before you have any tooth extraction or invasive dental procedure involving the jawbone.

85. Sclerostin inhibitors can cause _____. Report any swelling of the lips or rashes immediately.

CASE STUDY

Mrs. Laura Young is 60 years old. She began menopause at age 57. She is a moderate to heavy smoker. She has asked about HRT to relieve her menopause symptoms that have become more severe in the last few months. She has asked you about the risks and adverse side effects.

1. Which one of these risks for estrogen and progester-one drugs is greatly increased by smoking? (Choose the correct answer.)
   1. Myocardial infarction
   2. Excessive bleeding from the uterine lining
   3. The growth of hormone-sensitive cancers of the cervix, uterus, ovary, and breast
   4. Blood clotting and inappropriate development of thrombi and emboli

2. What can you teach Mrs. Young and her family about what they need to do during HRT treatment? (Check all that apply.)
   1. Take drugs for perimenopausal HRT exactly as prescribed with regard to dosage and timing.
   2. Quit or reduce smoking.
   3. Watch for salt craving, muscle weakness, hypo-tension, hypoglycemia (with headache, difficulty concentrating, shakiness), and fatigue.
   4. Check weekly for a yellow tinge on the roof of the mouth and whites of the eyes.
   5. Keep all appointments for laboratory blood work because these drugs alter blood levels of sodium and potassium.
   6. Take these drugs with food because they can cause nausea, vomiting, and other GI upsets.
   7. Call 911 immediately if you have chest pains, swelling in one leg, difficulty breathing, or signs of a stroke.
   8. Discuss the optimum length of time for treatment with your healthcare provider.

PRACTICE QUIZ

1. Bone density requires a constant supply of calcium. What supplement does dietary calcium need in order to be absorbed in the intestinal tract?
   a. Vitamin C
   b. Milk
   c. Estrogen
   d. Activated vitamin D

2. Given that strengths and types are varied for differ-ent brands of hormones, which hormone when pre-scribed cannot be exchanged for another brand?
   a. Adrenal hormones
   b. Thyroid hormone agonists and antithyroid hormones
   c. Perimenopausal HRT drugs and oral contraceptives
   d. Estrogen agonists/antagonists

3. Hypothyroidism can occur in children, even from birth. How long must a child with this disorder take thyroid hormone replacement drugs?
   a. Until the child reaches puberty
   b. At least 2 years
   c. Their entire life
   d. Until the child reaches 18 years of age

4. Thyroid hormone agonists are safe and necessary to use during pregnancy to protect the fetus. When can mothers being treated with thyroid hormone agonists not use this drug?
   a. During breastfeeding
   b. While taking oral contraceptives
   c. 1 month before delivery
   d. 2 months after delivery

5. Adults over 65 years are usually prescribed a lower initial dose of thyroid hormone agonists because they are more likely to have what effects?
   a. Nausea, dizziness, and vomiting
   b. Cushing's disease
   c. Blood clotting and edema
   d. Serious adverse cardiac and nervous system effects

6. How long must thyroid-suppressing drugs be taken before the patient starts to see an effect?
   a. 1 year
   b. 3 to 4 weeks
   c. 6 months
   d. 1 week

7. Which class of drugs cannot be taken during preg-nancy or breastfeeding?
   a. Thyroid hormone agonists
   b. Estrogen agonists/antagonists
   c. Antithyroid drugs
   d. Warfarin

107

8. Who are the drugs used to suppress adrenal hormone production not approved for?
   a. Patients over 65
   b. Patients under the age of 2
   c. Male patients
   d. Women who are pregnant or breastfeeding

9. The symptoms of menopause are caused by low levels of estrogen and high levels of what hormone?
   a. Follicle-stimulating hormone (FSH)
   b. Gonadotropin-releasing hormone (GNRH)
   c. Luteinizing hormone (LH)
   d. Progesterone

10. Which one of the following is not a symptom of hypothyroidism?
    a. Body temperature below normal
    b. Constipation
    c. Increased facial and body hair, decreased scalp hair
    d. Weight loss

11. What is the most common cause of hyperthyroidism?
    a. Goiter
    b. Basedow's disease
    c. Graves' disease
    d. Pretibial myxedema

12. What are the names of the two layers of the adrenal gland?
    a. Cortex and medulla
    b. Capsule and medulla
    c. Adrenal fat and the kidney
    d. Zona glomerulosa and zona reticularis

13. Mifepristone is only approved for patients with hypercortisolism and what other disease?
    a. Hyperaldosteronism
    b. Type 2 diabetes
    c. Menstrual irregularities
    d. Hypoglycemia

14. What causes the hot flashes (hot flushes) with facial redness and feelings of overheating during menopause?
    a. The secretion of gonadotropin-releasing hormone (GnRH) in the brain
    b. The luteinizing hormone causing the ovary to secrete progesterone
    c. High levels of FSH acting on blood vessels to make them dilate suddenly
    d. Ovulation

15. What is the process that causes old bone cells to be continually removed from bones?
    a. Osteoblastic
    b. Osteoclastic
    c. Osteoporosis
    d. Menopause

18 Drug Therapy for Diabetes

TYPES OF DIABETES MELLITUS

For each of the statements below, indicate if it describes diabetes mellitus type 1 (1), diabetes mellitus type 2 (2), or both types 1 and 2 (B).

1. _____ Autoimmune disorder

2. _____ The pancreas continues to make some insulin

3. _____ Beta cells of pancreas that manage insulin have been destroyed

4. _____ Long-term complications can shorten the life span of the individual

5. _____ May not have to take insulin if controlled adequately

6. _____ Body's immune system creates antibodies against insulin-secreting cells in the pancreas

7. _____ Usually caused by genetic predisposition or exposure to certain viruses

8. _____ There is a reduced response to insulin, known as insulin resistance

9. _____ Frequently diagnosed in childhood

10. _____ Frequently caused by obesity and decreased physical activity

11. _____ The pancreas produces no insulin

12. _____ The patient must take insulin for the remainder of his or her life unless they receive a pancreas transplant

MATCHING

Match the drugs listed in the left column with the drug categories on the right.

Drugs

13. _____ Dulaglutide

14. _____ Canagliflozin

15. _____ NovoLog

16. _____ Humulin R

17. _____ Metformin

18. _____ Pioglitazone

19. _____ Glimepiride

20. _____ Saxagliptin

21. _____ Levemir

22. _____ Alogliptin

23. _____ Acarbose

24. _____ Second-generation sulfonylurea agents

25. _____ Empagliflozin

26. _____ Lixisenatide

27. _____ Pramlintide

Drug Categories

A. Insulin stimulators (secretogogues)
B. Biguanides
C. Insulin sensitizers
D. Alpha-glucosidase inhibitors
E. Incretin mimetics
F. Amylin analogs
G. DPP-4 inhibitors
H. Sodium-glucose cotransport inhibitors
I. Insulin

Match the term with the correct definition.

Definition

28. _____ is a condition of higher-than-normal blood glucose levels.

29. _____ is a protein hormone produced by the pancreas or injected as a drug that binds to insulin receptors on many cells, which then promotes the movement of glucose from the blood into the cells.

30. _____ is a condition of lower-than-normal blood glucose levels.

31. _____ is a common chronic endocrine problem in which either the lack of insulin or poor function of insulin impairs glucose metabolism and leads to problems in fat and protein metabolism.

32. _____ are a category of noninsulin antidiabetic drugs that lower blood glucose levels by preventing the kidney from reabsorbing glucose that was filtered from the blood into the urine. This glucose then remains in the urine and is excreted rather than moved back into the blood.

33. _____ are oral and injectable drugs that use a variety of mechanisms other than binding to insulin receptors to help lower blood glucose levels back to the normal range.

34. _____ is a category of noninsulin antidiabetic drugs that help prevent hyperglycemia by reducing the amount of the DPP-4, which inactivates the normal incretins GLP and GIP. This allows the naturally produced incretins to be present and work with insulin to control blood glucose levels.

35. _____ is an oral noninsulin antidiabetic drug that lowers blood glucose levels by preventing enzymes in the intestinal tract from breaking down starches and more complex sugars into glucose.

36. _____ is an injectable noninsulin antidiabetic drug similar to natural amylin, which is a hormone produced by pancreatic beta cells and is cosecreted with insulin in response to blood glucose elevation. It prevents hyperglycemia by delaying gastric emptying and making the patient feel full.

37. _____ is a category of noninsulin antidiabetic drug that acts like the natural gut hormones (e.g., GLP-1) that are secreted in response to food in the stomach. They work with insulin to prevent blood glucose levels from becoming too high after meals by slowing the rate of gastric emptying.

38. _____ is a sugar-based nutrient critically important for energy production in cells and organs.

39. _____ is an oral noninsulin antidiabetic drug that lowers blood glucose levels by reducing the glucose the liver releases and by reducing how much and how fast the intestines absorb the glucose in food.

40. _____ are a category of oral noninsulin antidiabetic drugs that lower blood glucose levels by making insulin receptors more sensitive to insulin, which increases cellular uptake and use of glucose.

41. _____ are a category of oral noninsulin antidiabetic drugs that lower blood glucose levels by triggering the release of insulin stored in the beta cells of the pancreas. The sulfonylureas and the meglitinides are the two classes of drugs in this category.

Term

A. Alpha-glucosidase inhibitors
B. Amylin analogs
C. Biguanides
D. Diabetes mellitus
E. DPP-4 inhibitors
F. Glucose
G. Hyperglycemia
H. Hypoglycemia
I. Incretin mimetics
J. Insulin
K. Insulin sensitizers
L. Insulin stimulators
M. Noninsulin antidiabetic drugs
N. Sodium-glucose cotransport inhibitors

110

SIDE AND ADVERSE EFFECTS OF DRUGS FOR DIABETES

42. Complete the table

CATEGORIES	SIDE EFFECTS	ADVERSE EFFECTS
Insulin stimulators	_____ _____ _____ _____ _____	Hypoglycemia Can cause the beta cells of the pancreas to stop producing insulin, a condition known as "secondary beta cell failure" Can affect the liver and increase liver enzyme levels
Biguanides	Nausea Diarrhea Flatulence Weight loss	_____ _____ _____ _____ _____
Insulin sensitizers	Hypoglycemia Headache Sneezing Sore throat	_____ _____ _____ _____ _____
Alpha-glucosidase inhibitors	_____ _____ _____ _____ _____	Inflammation of the bowel such as colitis Crohn's disease or intestinal obstruction Hypoglycemia Liver impairment with elevated liver enzyme levels
Incretin mimetics	Nausea, vomiting Diarrhea Upper respiratory tract symptoms Weight loss	_____ _____ _____ _____ _____
_____	Nausea Vomiting Headache Abdominal pain Weight loss and fatigue Dizziness	Severe hypoglycemia Pancreatitis

CATEGORIES	SIDE EFFECTS	ADVERSE EFFECTS
DPP-4 inhibitors	_____ _____ _____ _____ _____ _____ _____ _____ _____	Hypoglycemia Allergic reactions with symptoms of hives, facial swelling, and itching Acute and even fatal pancreatitis Severe arthralgia (joint pain) Bullous pemphigoid, a rare skin condition that results in large, fluid-filled blisters that most often occur in the lower abdomen, upper thighs, or armpits
Sodium-glucose Cotransport inhibitors	Increased need to urinate Because glucose is excreted in the urine, patients using glucose strips to check for glucose in the urine will see a positive result most of the time. Weight loss initially through the loss of fluid, followed by loss of fat mass	_____ _____ _____ _____ _____ _____ _____ _____ _____ _____ _____
_____	Mild allergic reactions such as swelling, itching, or redness around the injection site and changes to the skin at injection sites	Hypoglycemia leading to loss of consciousness and even death Injection site infections

MULTIPLE CHOICE

For each of the drug categories listed below, check all items that describe what should be taught to patients and families.

43. Insulin stimulators (secretogogues)

    a. _____ Take these drugs at least 2 hours before meals.

    b. _____ Hypoglycemia symptoms include hunger pangs, nervousness, confusion, and tremors.

    c. _____ Check with the healthcare provider before taking any over-the-counter or prescription drugs to ensure stabilized blood glucose levels.

    d. _____ Avoid exercise at least 4 hours after taking these drugs.

44. Biguanides

    a. _____ Avoid drinking alcohol, as this increases chance of developing lactic acidosis.

    b. _____ Common side effects include rashes, increased urine output, and headaches.

    c. _____ Check with healthcare providers about stopping and starting drugs if radiopaque dye is being used.

    d. _____ Laboratory tests are important due to risk of cardiovascular disease and B_{12} deficiency.

45. Insulin sensitizers

   a. _____ If you miss a dose, take as soon as possible and do not double dosages

   b. _____ Report any of the following to your healthcare provider: itching, hives, swelling, changes in vision, swelling of feet or angles, rapid weight gain, or symptoms of hyperglycemia.

   c. _____ Avoid alcohol, which can affect blood glucose levels

   d. _____ Avoid all foods with sugar if symptoms of hypoglycemia are present

   e. _____ Check your blood sugar on a monthly basis

   f. _____ Due to the FDA black box warnings these drugs should not be taken by patients who have symptomatic heart failure or other specific types of cardiovascular disease.

46. Alpha-glucosidase Inhibitors

   a. _____ When taking these drugs, you should avoid all exercise.

   b. _____ These drugs must be taken at the end of meals to get the most benefit.

   c. _____ The drug's effect on blood sugar levels following meals depends on the amount of protein in the meal.

   d. _____ Avoid alcohol while taking these drugs as they increase risk of liver impairment.

47. Incretin mimetics

   a. _____ If you have difficulty breathing, a lump in your throat, or swelling of your mouth and tongue, call 911.

   b. _____ Alcohol increases risk of pancreatic inflammation

   c. _____ If a dose is missed, double your next dosage

   d. _____ Administer subcutaneous injection in thigh, upper arm, or abdomen

   e. _____ Inject the drug 60 minutes *after* meals

48. Amylin analogs

   a. _____ Opened vials and injectable pens should be refrigerated or used within 28 days.

   b. _____ The drug should warm to room temperature before injecting.

   c. _____ Administer this drug right after your meal

   d. _____ Do not mix pramlintide with insulin in the same syringe

   e. _____ Dispose of all used syringes and needles in a plastic bag

   f. _____ Do not drive or operate machinery until you know whether this drug causes dizziness

49. DPP-4 inhibitors

   a. _____ If a dose is accidentally missed, do not double up on the subsequent drug dose

   b. _____ Report any hypoglycemia incidents to your healthcare provider

   c. _____ Report symptoms of allergic reaction, angioedema, or pancreatitis to your healthcare provider

   d. _____ These drugs are safe to use if you are pregnant or breastfeeding.

   e. _____ An increased risk for heart failure has been reported in patients receiving saxagliptin and alogliptin. Therefore, patients receiving these drugs should have their weight checked daily. Report a weight gain of 2 or more pounds in a day or the onset of shortness of breath.

50. Sodium-glucose cotransport Inhibitors

    a. _____ Check your blood sugar at regular intervals

    b. _____ Report any weight gain to your healthcare provider

    c. _____ Report signs of UTI or vaginal infection

    d. _____ Limit fluids throughout the day

    e. _____ Glucose will be present in your urine while taking this drug.

51. Insulin

    a. _____ When symptoms of hypoglycemia are present, avoid eating or drinking anything until the symptoms pass

    b. _____ When symptoms of hyperglycemia are present, eat or drink something containing sugar

    c. _____ Seek emergency treatment for symptoms of ketoacidosis

    d. _____ Keep appointments with your healthcare provider to test your blood glucose levels

    e. _____ Insulin vials must be stored at room temperature

    f. _____ Shake insulin vials vigorously before drawing the insulin up

    g. _____ Avoid alcohol because it can intensify hypoglycemia

    h. _____ Carry a readily available source of protein at all times in case you develop symptoms of hypoglycemia

GIVING INSULIN WITH A PEN DEVICE

52. Fill in the missing steps.
    a. Wash your hands.
    b. Check the order and the drug label.
    c. Remove the cap.
    d. _____
    e. Wipe the tip of the pen where the needle will attach with an alcohol swab.
    f. _____
    g. Remove both the plastic outer cap and inner needle cap.
    h. _____
    i. Holding the pen with the needle pointing upward, press the button until at least a drop of insulin appears. This is the "cold shot," "air shot," or "safety shot." Repeat this step if needed until a drop appears.
    j. _____
    k. Hold the pen perpendicular to and press against the injection site with your thumb on the dosing knob.
    l. _____
    m. Hold the pen in place for 6 to 10 seconds; then withdraw from the skin.
    n. Replace the outer needle cap, unscrew until the needle is removed, and dispose of the needle in a hard plastic or metal container.
    o. _____

CASE STUDY

Mr. Antwan Spears is a 69-year-old Native American male who has a 5-year history of type 2 diabetes. Mr. Spears arrives at his primary care provider's office for a follow-up examination. His physician is concerned because of his family history of type 2 diabetes, heart disease, and stroke. Mr. Spears states his fasting blood glucose levels are 185 to 220 mg/dL. He also states he has been adherent to his meal plan and has been taking walks more often to increase his activity level. He presents at the examination with dizziness, shakiness, sweatiness, and confusion. He has been using nateglinide (Starlix) 120 mg orally three times daily with meals. From the information you gathered so far, it is unclear why Mr. Spears is hypoglycemic.

1. In addition to dizziness, shakiness, sweatiness, and confusion, what are other symptoms of hypoglycemia that you should teach to Mr. Spears? (Choose all that apply.)
    1. Headache
    2. Hunger sensation
    3. Difficulty concentrating
    4. Nervousness and anxiety
    5. Fruity-smelling breath
    6. Frequent urination
    7. Pale, clammy skin
    8. Rapid heart rate
    9. Nausea and vomiting

2. After questioning Mr. Spears further, you find out he has been regularly taking ibuprofen for joint pain. What other drugs interact with nateglinide (Starlix) that might cause hypoglycemia?
   1. Aspirin and other nonsteroidal antiinflammatories (NSAIDs)
   2. Angiotensin II receptor antagonists (ARBs)
   3. Pseudoephedrine
   4. Angiotensin converting enzyme inhibitors (ACEIs)
   5. Beta-blockers
   6. Antiretroviral protease inhibitors
   7. Warfarin
   8. Azole antifungal drugs
   9. Thiazide diuretics
   10. Many antibiotics
   11. Corticosteroids

PRACTICE QUIZ

1. What is the purpose of glucose, a sugar-based nutrient?
   a. Binds insulin receptors on many cells
   b. Metabolizes within the cells to generate the body's energy
   c. Prevents hyperglycemia
   d. Released within the body when energy is low

2. How does insulin, a protein hormone produced by the pancreas, prevent hyperglycemia?
   a. Provides the muscles with energy
   b. Prevents the body from storing sugar
   c. Prevents the kidney from eliminating glucose
   d. Allows body cells to take up, use, and store carbohydrate, fat, and protein

3. How does glucagon work to prevent low blood glucose levels?
   a. Triggers the release of glucose from the liver and skeletal muscle when blood glucose is lower than normal
   b. Prevents the release of insulin from the pancreas when blood glucose is lower than normal
   c. Protects cells from releasing too much energy when blood glucose is lower than normal
   d. Ensures sufficient insulin is released from the pancreas when blood glucose is lower than normal

4. Why do the neurons and the brain require a continuous supply of glucose from the blood?
   a. The brain and neurons are continuously working to keep the body functioning.
   b. The brain stores only a minimal amount of fat which must be continuously replenished.
   c. The brain is unable to store any glucose.
   d. The brain and neurons use significantly more glucose than other parts of the body.

5. What is the primary cause of diabetes mellitus?
   a. An overproduction of insulin which inhibits glucose from functioning adequately
   b. Glucose is not released in adequate amounts into the bloodstream.
   c. The brain and neurons do not receive an adequate supply of glucose and therefore the organs began not operating efficiently.
   d. Glucose movement from the blood into cells and organs is impaired.

6. What are some of the complications of uncontrolled/poorly controlled diabetes mellitus?
   a. Sterility
   b. Restrictions in activities
   c. Reduced functions of all organs and tissues
   d. Blood pressure lower than normal

7. What causes the potentially fatal condition known as ketoacidosis?
   a. A patient with diabetes mellitus eats an excess of protein.
   b. The body uses stored fat for energy in place of glucose.
   c. The pancreas creates an excess of insulin, causing the body to use muscle protein for energy in place of glucose.
   d. A patient with diabetes mellitus drinks an excess of alcohol.

8. While type 1 diabetes onset is sudden and severe and quickly diagnosed, why is type 2 diabetes usually not diagnosed as quickly?
   a. Type 2 diabetes is only diagnosed if blood glucose levels are tested regularly.
   b. Because in type 2 diabetes the pancreas still produces some insulin, symptoms may not occur until complications begin.
   c. In some individuals, type 2 diabetes symptoms may eventually dissipate over time.
   d. Type 2 diabetes often presents as pancreatitis and the other symptoms are overlooked.

9. When a patient is first diagnosed with type 2 diabetes, what is the best first line of treatment for the chronic disease?
   a. Insulin injections to replace the levels no longer produced by the pancreas
   b. Non-insulin antidiabetic drugs to control blood glucose levels
   c. No treatment is recommended until consistent testing of blood glucose levels indicates a consistent, higher-than-normal level.
   d. Patients should try diet and exercise first to determine if those measures will help them maintain a target blood glucose level.

115

10. What is necessary for insulin-stimulator oral drugs to lower blood glucose levels?
    a. The patient must take the drug consistently on a daily basis to ensure effectiveness.
    b. The patient must have some functioning beta cells within the pancreas.
    c. The patient must have a blood glucose level that is closer to normal range.
    d. The patient must maintain a healthy diet and program of exercise.

11. What is the only drug available in the biguanides category of drugs?
    a. Metformin
    b. Miglitol
    c. Exenatide
    d. Saxagliptin

12. Which category of drug is most often recommended for patients who have high blood sugar following meals?
    a. Insulin sensitizers
    b. Alpha-glucosidase inhibitors
    c. Incretin mimetics
    d. Amylin analogs

13. Where should subcutaneous injections be administered?
    a. Rotate between upper arm and upper thigh
    b. Rotate between both sides of lower abdomen
    c. Select upper arm, upper thigh, or abdomen and consistently use the same location
    d. Rotate among upper arm, upper thigh, and abdomen

14. What is considered a normal fasting blood glucose level?
    a. 70 to 90 mg/dL
    b. 60 to 100 mg/dL
    c. 75 to 115 mg/dL
    d. 80 to 90 mg/dL

15. Why should insulin be administered by the parenteral route?
    a. Because insulin must be refrigerated, it can upset the stomach.
    b. It is necessary to use a faster route of administration for insulin.
    c. Because insulin is destroyed by stomach acids and intestinal enzymes
    d. Prevents stress on the pancreas

19 | Drugs for Eye and Ear Problems

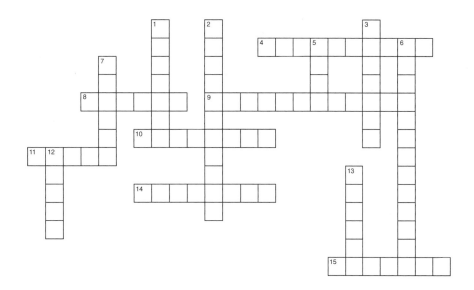

ACROSS

4. Carries messages from the special cells in the retina to the brain, where we then "see" the images
8. Stirrups
9. The watery fluid that fills the space between the cornea and the lens
10. Three small bones in the middle ear
11. The external ear
14. The S-shaped tube leading from the pinna to the ear drum
15. Tympanic membrane

DOWN

1. Hammer
2. Normal circulation of the watery fluid maintains a normal _____ pressure (IOP).
3. Ear wax
5. Muscular ring around the eye
6. Jellylike substance that fills the posterior segment of the eye
7. Lining of the back of the eye
12. Anvil
13. Clear covering of the eye that allows light to enter

KEY TERMS

Match terms to the correct description.

Descriptions

16. _____ Liquid or ointment drugs prepared to place on the eye or the conjunctiva

17. _____ Drugs that bind to specific prostaglandin receptor sites in the eye, causing an increase outflow of aqueous humor

18. _____ These drugs bind to receptor sites in the eye and reduce the amount of aqueous humor produced

19. _____ A type of diuretic that also can lower intraocular pressure by decreasing production of aqueous humor by 50–60%

20. _____ Drugs that increase the availability of acetylcholine to activate specific receptors. This leads to decreased production of aqueous humor and improved outflow of aqueous humor to decrease intraocular pressure.

21. _____ Drugs that soften ear wax

22. _____ Drugs that inhibit adrenergic receptor sites in the eye and decrease production of aqueous humor

23. _____ Drugs prepared for delivery into the external ear canal

Terms

A. Alpha-adrenergic agonists
B. Beta-adrenergic blocking agents
C. Carbonic anhydrase inhibitors (CAIs)
D. Cerumenolytics
E. Cholinergic agents
F. Ophthalmic drugs
G. Otic drugs
H. Prostaglandin agonists

EAR PROBLEMS (Fill in the Blanks)

24. The most common ear problems that occur in the external ear and in the middle ear are _____ and _____.

25. When these problems occur in the middle ear, _____ and _____ are given systemically, most often by the oral route.

26. When these common ear problems occur in the pinna and the ear canal, they are most often managed by _____ drug application.

27. Drugs that are prepared to apply into the external ear canal are _____ drugs.

28. The length and angle of ear canals differ between young children and adults. In adults, the ear canal tilts downward, is longer, and is slightly curved in an S-shape. In children, the canal is shorter and straighter. These differences require distinct techniques when instilling otic drugs.

    Adults: _____

    _____

    Children: _____

    _____

29. What symptoms may occur with excessive wax buildup in the ear?

    _____

    _____

30. Name the type of drugs that soften ear wax and can be instilled before irrigation.

_____

31. Never place a drug into the ear canal or irrigate the ear canal if there is _____ present because it could enter the middle ear and cause an infection. Also, do not place drugs into the ear canal if the patient is dizzy, as dizziness will be increased.

32. Number in correct order the steps for instilling topical drugs into the patient's ear canal.
    ☐ Wash hands and don a pair of clean gloves
    ☐ Remind the patient to keep the head in this position for 2 to 3 minutes to allow the drops to flow
    ☐ Read the label of the drug carefully to ensure that it is for "otic" use. Never put any solution in the ear that is not labeled specifically for use in ears.
    ☐ Warm the ear drops to room temperature
    ☐ For an older child or adult, pull the pinna up and back
    ☐ Using the applicator, place only the prescribed number of drops into the patient's ear. Aim the drops onto the side of the ear canal and let them run into the ear.
    ☐ Remove your gloves and wash hands
    ☐ Make sure that the patient's eardrum is intact. This may require assessment by the RN or other healthcare provider. Never give an ear drug if there is damage to the eardrum.
    ☐ Insert a cotton ball into the opening of the ear canal to keep the drops from rolling out of the ear
    ☐ For a young child (younger than 3), gently pull the pinna down and back
    ☐ Ask the patient to lie down with the head turned so that the affected eye is turned upward; if the patient is sitting in a chair, tilt the patient's head so the affected ear is up
    ☐ Verify the drug using the 9 rights of drug administration

EYE PROBLEMS (Fill in the Blanks)

33. Problems that affect the eyes and vision that can be managed with drug therapy are _____, _____, and _____.

34. Drugs for these problems are _____ drugs, which come in liquid drops or ointment form to place on the eye or the conjunctiva.

35. Pupil constriction is _____ (small word, small pupil size). Pupil dilation is _____ (larger word, larger pupil size).

36. Most _____ and _____ drugs used to treat eye problems have an ophthalmic form that can be administered topically.

37. Number in order the steps for administering eye drops or ointments to a patient.
    ☐ Without pressing on the eyelid, gently blot or wipe away any excess drug or tears with a tissue.
    ☐ Wash your hands and put on gloves.
    ☐ Wash your hands again.
    ☐ Replace contact lenses as appropriate.
    ☐ Remove your gloves.
    ☐ Remind the patient that his or her vision will be blurry and not to drive until the vision clears.
    ☐ Recap the tube or bottle.
    ☐ Make sure the patient is not wearing contact lenses; if they are, ask the patient to remove them.
    ☐ If both eyes are to receive the same drug and one eye is infected, use two separate bottles or tubes and carefully label each with "right" or "left" for the correct eye.
    ☐ Hold the eye-drop bottle or ointment tube (with the cap off) like a pencil, with the tip pointing down.
    ☐ Have the patient sit in a chair while you stand behind the patient (or alternatively, stand in front of the patient, who is sitting in a chair or over the patient who is lying in bed).
    ☐ Gently release the lower lid.
    ☐ Gently pull the lower lid down against the patient's cheek, forming a small pocket.

☐ For ointment, squeeze a small amount out onto a tissue (without touching the tip to the tissue) and discard this ointment.

☐ For eye drops, with a gloved finger, gently press and hold the corner of the eye nearest the nose to close off the tear duct and prevent the drug from being absorbed systemically.

☐ For eye drops, gently squeeze the bottle and release the prescribed number of drops into the pocket that you have made with the patient's lower eyelid. Do not touch any part of the eye or lid with the tip of the bottle. For ointment, gently squeeze the tube and release a small amount of ointment into the pocket that you have made with the patient's lower eye lid. Do not touch any part of the eye or lid with the tip of the tube.

☐ Explain the procedure to the patient.

☐ Check to see whether only one eye is to have the drug or if both eyes are to receive the drug.

☐ Check the name, strength, expiration date, color, and clarity of the eye drops to be instilled. If the drug is an ointment, be sure that it is an ophthalmic (eye) preparation and not a general topical ointment.

☐ Ask the patient to tilt the head backward, with the back of the head resting against you (or the back of the chair) and look up at the ceiling.

☐ Ask the patient to close the eye gently, without squeezing the lids tightly, and roll the eye under the lid to spread the drug across the eye for about 2 minutes.

GLAUCOMA (Fill in the Blanks)

38. Glaucoma is a chronic eye disease of increased _____ pressure that causes damage to the optic nerve.

39. If untreated, glaucoma causes loss of _____ and even blindness.

40. Glaucoma is an eye disorder resulting from too much _____.

41. Name the most common type of glaucoma.

_____ (POAG)

42. Drug therapy for patients with glaucoma involves _____ the amount of aqueous humor produced by the ciliary body or improving drainage and reabsorption of the aqueous humor. This decreases fluid pressure in the eye and relieves pressure on the _____ and the _____.

120

Match the glaucoma drugs with the corresponding action, uses, side effects, and possible adverse reactions. Each drug will be used more than once.

Corresponding Actions

43. _____ Systemic absorption may cause adverse reactions such as changes in blood pressure and abnormal heart rhythms. Other adverse effects include double vision and retinal detachment.

44. _____ Related to sulfonamide drugs and may cause an allergic reaction in patients allergic to any sulfa drug. Oral or IV administration can cause confusion, dizziness, numbness of the hands and feet, even paralysis, severe skin infections, severe electrolyte imbalances, and liver failure

45. _____ Help control glaucoma by binding to receptor sites in the eye and relax eye blood vessel smooth muscles, which allows these blood vessels to dilate and absorb aqueous humor

46. _____ Expected side effects of this class of drugs include tearing, stinging, redness of the eye, blurred vision, and mitosis. Systemic side effects are possible and include headache, increased salivation, increased urination, and sweating.

47. _____ Adverse effects may be bradycardia or tachycardia and a drop in blood pressure. Also, there may be allergic reaction, fatigue, and respiratory symptoms.

48. _____ Decreases IOP by reducing the amount of aqueous humor produced and improving its flow. By increasing the amount of this drug, the pupil becomes smaller (miosis). This in turn increases the amount of space between the lens and the iris, allowing the aqueous fluid to flow freely, decreasing IOP.

49. _____ Side effects include temporary blurring of vision, slight burning or stinging, and tearing of the eye. Later, the patient may notice less tear production and dry, itchy, or red eyes. Pupils will not dilate as easily when entering a dark room.

50. _____ Reduces the amount of aqueous humor produced from the ciliary body of the eye

51. _____ Lower IOP by reducing aqueous humor in the anterior chamber of the eye This class of drugs is a type of diuretic.

52. _____ Slight burning or stinging with administration Some patients may experience a bitter or sour taste in the mouth. In rare cases, redness of the conjunctiva can occur.

53. _____ If absorbed systemically, this class of drug can cause decreased heart rate, decreased blood pressure, and even heart failure. Systemic absorption can also cause bronchoconstriction and asthma symptoms.

54. _____ Can rarely experience infection, asthma, and corneal erosion (damage to the cornea).

55. _____ Class of drug that acts to reduce the amount of aqueous humor produced in the eye. In addition, they improve the flow of aqueous humor out of the anterior chamber of the eye.

56. _____ Causes eye itching and eye redness when first applied. Patients can have a foreign body sensation. The iris color may change to brown, lashes may thicken and lengthen, and dark skin may appear under the eye.

57. _____ Tearing, redness, blurring of vision and burning, stinging or sensation of foreign object after giving the eye drops are common side effects.

Drugs

A. Alpha-adrenergic agonists
B. Beta-adrenergic blocking agents
C. Anhydrase inhibitors (CAIs)
D. Cholinergic agents
E. Prostaglandin agonists

Chapter **19 Drugs for Eye and Ear Problems**

58. Why is it not advisable to use higher than prescribed doses of prostaglandin agonist?

    _____

59. When using prostaglandin agonists, if you have lighter-colored eyes, what three things can change over time?

    a. _____   b. _____

    c. _____

60. If you have glaucoma only in one eye, prostaglandin agonist drops should be placed in both eyes so the colors will match. True or False? _____

61. Do not increase the dose of beta-adrenergic antagonists or use the drug more often because excessive use increases the risk for _____

    _____

62. When using beta-adrenergic antagonists or cholinergic drugs, why should good lighting always be used?

    _____

    _____

63. If you have diabetes, check your blood glucose more often because beta-adrenergic antagonists can _____ of hypoglycemia if the drug is absorbed systemically.

64. When giving beta-adrenergic antagonists to older patients, make sure they are not taking any _____ drugs for a cardiac condition. If so, notify the healthcare provider. Older adults are more likely to have cardiac and respiratory problems from systemic absorption of eye drops.

65. Make sure to read packaging carefully, as some alpha-adrenergic drugs may need to be stored in the _____ and _____ to maintain potency.

66. If being treated with alpha-adrenergic drugs, wear dark glasses when you are in the sunlight or other bright light conditions because your pupil will be _____ and your eye will be sensitive to the light.

67. If you have been prescribed an alpha-adrenergic drug for a limited time, such as 1 week, do not continue the drug beyond that time period. Explain why this is true.

    _____

68. Give the main reason for immediately wiping up any spills of cholinergic drops from the patient's skin. _____

    _____

69. What two symptoms indicate a toxic level of cholinergic drugs and should be reported to a healthcare provider immediately?

    a. _____

    b. _____

70. Do not give carbonic anhydrase inhibitors (CAIs) to _____ and avoid during _____ and _____.

71. After giving eye drops, ask the patient to close his or her eyes for _____. This reduces the amount of drug absorbed systemically. A second option to reduce systemic absorption of the drug is to apply gentle pressure with the index finger over the _____ for about 3 minutes after giving the eye drops.

122

CASE STUDY

Mr. Sam Collins is an 80-year-old man who presents with reduced hearing and ear pain. He has been told it is normal for his age to have reduced hearing and has not received any treatment for his condition. Upon examination, you find he has impacted ear wax (cerumen) that may be causing his hearing loss and pain. You suggest a **cerumenolytic drug** (to soften ear wax) to be instilled before irrigating the ear canal.

1. What do you need to teach Mr. Collins about using a cerumenolytic drug? (Choose all that apply.)
   1. These drugs are available over the counter and can be used at home by the patient. Make sure the drops say for optic use only.
   2. An antifungal or antimicrobial drug can be taken orally first to loosen the ear wax if it is impacted deeply.
   3. Remember to teach patients to *never* use it in an ear that has drainage or discharge
   4. Mr. Collins should be referred to an audiologist for a hearing test.
   5. Do not instill a cerumenolytic or irrigate an ear canal in a person who is dizzy.
   6. Recent literature suggests that distilled water or saline may be just as effective as oil- or peroxide-based solutions.
   7. Mr. Collins can go to a specialist to remove the impacted ear wax if instilling the cerumenolytic drug and irrigation does not help.

2. What can you teach Mr. Collins about the correct way to instill the cerumenolytic ear drops?
   1. Pull the external ear up and back.
   2. Pull the external ear down and back.

Susan Armstrong is a 55-year-old woman who was recently diagnosed with glaucoma in her right eye. The diagnosis was identified during a routine eye exam. To control the glaucoma, her healthcare provider prescribes Lumigan, a prostaglandin agonist. These types of drugs relax eye blood vessel smooth muscles, which allows these blood vessels to dilate and absorb aqueous humor.

3. What can you do to help Susan use the drug correctly? (Select all that apply.)
   1. Check Susan's eye for scratches or trauma.
   2. Recommend regular eyebrow grooming to ensure cleanliness around the eye.
   3. Recommend that Susan look for darker colors on her eyelid.
   4. Let Susan know she may notice changes in the color of the affected eye.
   5. If an eyelash falls into the affected eye, Susan should use the medication to wash it out of her eye.
   6. Susan should abstain from alcohol and cannabis to reduce eye pressure.
   7. Inform her not to use in unaffected eye to make the lashes grown longer and thicker.
   8. Warn Susan that when first using the drops, she may feel as if something is in her eye.

PRACTICE QUIZ

1. Cerumenolytic drugs are sold over the counter and usually contain what chemical?
   a. Apraclonidine
   b. Brinzolamide
   c. Carbamide peroxide
   d. Carbastat

2. Aqueous humor is produced by which part of the eye?
   a. Retina
   b. Ciliary body
   c. Optic nerve
   d. Lacrimal gland

3. What is the normal intraocular pressure of the eye?
   a. 10 to 20 mm Hg
   b. 30 to 40 mm Hg
   c. 32 psi
   d. 120/80 to 140/90

4. Which institute provides an excellent Internet resource for healthcare professionals, patients, and families about various eye disorders, with information and photographs?
   a. The Johns Hopkins Wilmer Eye Institute (www.hopkinsmedicine.org/wilmer)
   b. The National Eye Institute (NEI) (https://nei.nih.gov/)
   c. The Vanderbilt Eye Institute (https://www.vanderbilthealth.com/eyeinstitute/)
   d. Rand Eye Institute (https://www.randeye.com/about-us/)

5. Why is glaucoma called a "thief in the night" disease?
   a. The patient typically has no symptoms other than a gradual loss of peripheral side vision.
   b. The patient often has night blindness as a first symptom.
   c. The patient has sudden loss of vision.
   d. The patient only experiences symptoms when first waking up in the morning.

6. What is the rare type of glaucoma that causes a sudden increase of intraocular pressure and patient experiences severe headache, nausea, and vomiting, and a halo effect around lights?
   a. Primary open angle
   b. Secondary closed angle
   c. Acute open angle
   d. Acute angle closure

7. Under what circumstances should you never instill prostaglandin agonists in a patient's eye?
   a. Headaches and sinus congestion
   b. Scratches or infection
   c. Dark coloring under the eye
   d. Pupil is dilated

123

8. What suffix (word ending) do beta-blockers have?
   a. "ine"
   b. "mide"
   c. "olol"
   d. "mic"

9. Patients with glaucoma may have unequal size of what part of the eye? If this situation exists, you should consult with patient's healthcare provider.
   a. Iris
   b. Eyelid
   c. Retina
   d. Pupil

10. What sudden changes related to cholinergic drugs should be reported to a healthcare provider immediately?
    a. Nausea and vomiting
    b. Blood pressure, heart rate, and difficulty breathing
    c. Anxiety
    d. Iris color changes to brown

11. Carbonic anhydrase inhibitors should not be given to patients with what condition?
    a. Sulfa allergy
    b. Diabetes
    c. Glaucoma
    d. Food allergies

12. Though rare, what side effects are possible with cerumenolytics?
    a. Loss of hearing for 2 to 3 minutes
    b. Popping sounds in the ear
    c. Redness, itching or rash
    d. Burning sensation in the ear canal

13. What patient action will provide maximum effectiveness of treatment when given cerumenolytics?
    a. A warm, moist cloth placed over the ear
    b. Heating the drops before administration
    c. Cooling the drops before administration
    d. Remain lying down for 5 minutes for optimum absorption

14. What should a patient be taught to do if there is a sudden decrease or loss of vision during ophthalmic drug therapy?
    a. Remain lying down until vision returns
    b. Rinse eyes with water or saline solution
    c. Call 911 or go to the nearest emergency room
    d. Contact their healthcare provider

15. What is the usual time period of drug therapy for glaucoma?
    a. 2 to 6 months
    b. The rest of the patient's life
    c. 3 weeks
    d. Until peripheral vision is restored

20 Over-the-Counter Drug Therapy

OVER-THE-COUNTER (OTC) DRUGS

(True or False)

1. _____ Instruct the patient to always read the instructions and possible side effects of OTC drugs from a reliable Internet source.

2. _____ OTC drugs and supplements, as opposed to prescription drugs, are safer and can be taken in higher doses and for longer periods of time than the instructions suggest.

3. _____ Because they are created to treat specific symptoms there are no adverse interactions between OTC drugs and other drugs the patient may be taking, food and alcohol, or other medical conditions the patient has.

4. _____ A pharmacist can be consulted if the patient is unsure about side effects of OTC drugs.

5. _____ Responses to the drugs vary from person to person.

6. _____ The patient should be informed that it is more cost effective and safer to buy OTC drugs online.

7. _____ To avoid poisoning, a parent should give children one-half the adult dose.

8. _____ Always follow the age limits listed. If the label says the product should not be given to a child younger than 2 years, then do not give it.

9. _____ Generic OTC drugs are often less expensive than brand names of the same drug.

10. _____ Drugs should be discarded if they are past the expiration date and if the packaging or instructions are missing.

11. _____ Because they are not prescriptions written expressly for the patient, OTC drugs can be used by other family members or friends with similar symptoms.

12. _____ Giving a child a drug containing alcohol is acceptable as they are not taking as high a dose as an adult.

13. _____ Always use the child-resistant cap and store drugs away from children.

14. _____ It is advisable to purchase OTC drugs that are multipurpose and which therefore may treat other symptoms as well as those the patient has.

(Fill in the blanks)

15. What is the website for educating your patients and yourself with current evidence-based research on various alternative drug therapies? _____

16. How do the FDA regulations differ for dietary supplements and prescription/OTC drugs?

    _____

    _____

    _____

    _____

17. If a dietary supplement is unsafe or ineffective, the FDA must prove this with scientific-based evidence. What is a supplement that was banned by the agency because it caused heart problems and other serious side effects when combined with caffeine?

    _____

18. What is the major criticism of herbal supplements?

    _____

    _____

    _____

    _____

19. What are three phytoestrogens promoted as a 'natural' therapy for menopause and hormone replacement that have not been proven to be any more effective than conventional hormone therapies?

    _____   _____   _____

20. Name three herbal products that are most likely to cause dangerous interactions with any prescription drugs the patient may be taking.

    _____   _____   _____

21. Calcium derived from oyster shells can contain what three dangerous substances?

    _____   _____   _____

22. Name the ways cannabis can be administered for medical treatment.

    _____ _____ _____ _____ _____

23. What conditions may CBD be useful to treat?

    _____ _____ _____ _____ _____

VITAMINS

Match the name of the vitamin with description of actions and deficiencies. Each vitamin will be used more than once.

24. _____ Important for vision, gene characteristics, reproduction, embryo growth and development, healthy immune system function, used to treat celiac, colitis, specific eye diseases and night blindness

25. _____ Water soluble and functions as a coenzyme in the metabolism of protein, carbohydrates, and fat

26. _____ Antiseizure drugs reduce the levels of this vitamin and sulfasalazine prevents intestinal absorption of it

27. _____ Assists in formation of blood formatting factors

28. _____ Promotes formation of collagen, healing, and absorption of iron

29. _____ Helps absorption of calcium and phosphorus

30. _____ Deficiency of this vitamin causes pellagra

31. _____ Deficiency of this vitamin causes pernicious anemia

32. _____ Prevents damage to cell membranes

33. _____ Deficiency causes B_6 anemia

34. _____ Controls amino acid metabolism and energy release

35. _____ Synthesizes DNA and supports RBC maturation

36. _____ Deficiency causes difficulty eating and swallowing

37. _____ Deficiency causes beriberi

38. _____ Helps formulate red blood cells

39. _____ Controls metabolism of CHO, protein, and fats

40. _____ Deficiency can cause scurvy

41. _____ Deficiency may cause rickets, osteomalacia, hypoparathyroidism

42. _____ Important for the metabolism of carbohydrates

43. _____ Deficiency causes blood clotting disorders

44. _____ Deficiency causes folic acid anemia

Vitamin A
Vitamin D
Vitamin E
Vitamin K
Vitamin B_{12}
Vitamin B_9
Vitamin B_3
Vitamin B_6
Vitamin B_2
Vitamin B_1

127

45. Name the primary food sources for each vitamin.

Vitamin A	Vitamin D
Vitamin E	Vitamin K
Vitamin B_{12}	Vitamin B_3
Vitamin B_9	Vitamin B_6
Vitamin B_1	Vitamin B_2

FILL IN THE BLANKS

46. What are the four signs of vitamin A overdose? _____

_____ _____ _____

47. _____ in food is destroyed if food is boiled, fried, or baked for a long time under pressure.

48. Give the alternate name for the B vitamins.

B_{12} _____ B_9 _____

B_3 _____ B_6 _____

B_1 _____ B_2 _____

49. If niacin is taken along with some hypertension drugs, a condition called _____ may occur. Patient should be told to sit or lie down if dizziness occurs.

50. Warn patients that taking riboflavin supplements can cause urine to become _____.

51. Name the three major forms of vitamin C.

_____ _____ _____

52. Give the therapeutic daily dose of vitamin D supplementation for the following two conditions:

Rickets _____

Hypoparathyroidism _____

53. _____ is the antidote for warfarin (Coumadin) overdose.

MINERALS

Match the name of the mineral with the description of uses, side effects or precautions.
Each mineral may be used more than once.

54. _____ Major mineral in the body and is essential for muscular and neurologic activity, especially in the cardiac system

55. _____ Part of many enzymes and is essential for normal growth and tissue repair. It functions in the mineralization of bone and in the detoxification of methanol and ethylene glycol. It plays a role in the creation of DNA and the synthesis of protein from amino acids. It is important in wound healing and functions in moving vitamin A from liver stores.

56. _____ Principal intracellular positive ion (*cation*) of most body tissues, acting in the maintenance of normal kidney function, contraction of muscle, and transmission of nerve impulses

57. _____ Slight deficiencies may prolong the Q-T interval and lead to an extremely dangerous form of *ventricular tachycardia* (rapid heartbeat) called *torsades de pointes*

58. _____ Essential mineral for the body to make myoglobin and hemoglobin

59. _____ Electrolyte that is essential to several enzyme systems. It is important in maintaining osmotic pressure, ion balance, bone structure, muscular contraction, and nerve conduction.

60. _____ Both low and high levels of this mineral can cause fatal heart arrhythmias

61. _____ Expected reactions to supplements of this mineral include constipation and cramping. Adverse reactions such as diarrhea, epigastric or abdominal pain may occur.

62. _____ Adverse reactions supplements of this mineral include gastric ulceration, nausea, and vomiting. Doses in excess of 2 g produce *emesis* (vomiting).

A. Calcium
B. Iron
C. Potassium
D. Magnesium
E. Zinc

63. _____ is essential for absorption of calcium.

64. Acute _____ intoxication produces drowsiness, lethargy, lightheadedness, staggering gait, restlessness, and vomiting leading to dehydration.

65. Signs of _____ are muscle spasms, numbness and tingling of the lips and fingers, weak and brittle nails, and fractures. Symptoms of _____ are polyuria (excretion of a large amount of urine), constipation, abdominal pain, dryness of mouth, anorexia, nausea, and vomiting.

66. Fatal anaphylactic reactions can occur with _____ IV or IM administration. Hypersensitivity reactions include rash, itching, joint pain, muscle aches, and fever.

67. Describe *Trousseau's sign.* _____

_____

_____

68. More _____ is absorbed if taken on an empty stomach or acid environment, while taking it with meals reduces irritation and absorption.

69. Deficiency of _____ may cause convulsions, slowing of growth, digestive disturbances, spasticity of muscles and nerves, accelerated heartbeat, dysrhythmias, nervous conditions, and vasodilation (opening of blood vessels).

70. All _____ supplements must be diluted properly or taken with plenty of liquid to avoid producing GI ulcers.

71. Patients should be advised that taking iron supplements causes _____. Tell patients to report constipation, diarrhea, nausea, or abdominal pain to the healthcare provider.

72. List food sources for the following minerals:

Calcium

Zinc

Iron

Magnesium

Potassium

CASE STUDY

A 62-year-old female patient has been receiving chemotherapy for ovarian cancer. She comes to the clinic for her routine bloodwork and lab results show her magnesium levels are low (1.2 mg/dL).

1. In addition to recommending a diet of foods that are rich in magnesium, you should tell the patient to avoid alcohol consumption. Why is this necessary? (Choose the correct answer.)
   1. Alcohol will impair the patient's judgment when choosing foods that provide magnesium.
   2. Lab results will be inconclusive if alcohol is present in the patient's blood.
   3. Alcohol use causes an increase in magnesium excretion by the kidneys and body stores of magnesium can be dangerously depleted with the chronic use of alcohol.
   4. Alcohol use while receiving chemotherapy can cause it to be ineffective.

2. What are the symptoms the patient may present with if there is a magnesium deficiency? (Select all that apply.)
   1. Torsades de pointes
   2. Convulsions
   3. Diarrhea
   4. Slowing of growth
   5. Digestive disturbances
   6. Anemia
   7. Spasticity of muscles and nerves
   8. Pale skin
   9. Accelerated heartbeat
   10. Dysrhythmias
   11. Numbness and tingling
   12. Nervous conditions
   13. Vasodilation

Mary Smith has been struggling with anxiety and repeatedly presents at your clinic for help with various complaints. Eventually, the health care provider recognizes that anxiety is Mary's principal problem and prescribes Xanax.

3. At first, Mary seems to be calmer while taking the Xanax, but after several months, the medicine no longer seems to be as effective. You do a history with Mary. Which of the following items can indicate why the Xanax is not as effective?
   1. Mary does not exercise regularly.
   2. Mary has problems with her family.
   3. Mary takes St. John's wort to help with her anxiety.
   4. Mary smokes regularly.

PRACTICE QUIZ

1. Which of the vitamins most commonly prescribed for supplementation are fat soluble?
   a. A, C, E, and K
   b. A, D, E, and K
   c. A, B_{12}, D, and E
   d. C, E, D, and K

2. An excess of vitamin A during pregnancy can cause birth defects in which of the baby's systems?
   a. Digestive
   b. Endocrine
   c. Central nervous
   d. Exocrine

3. What hidden drug is found in many cough syrups, cold medications, and mouthwashes?
   a. Caffeine
   b. Sodium
   c. Magnesium
   d. Alcohol

4. Which vitamin, when administered parenterally, can cause allergic reactions including feelings of warmth, pruritus, urticaria, nausea, angioedema, shortness of breath, sweating, tightness of the throat, and cyanosis?
   a. Thiamin
   b. Niacin
   c. Beta-carotene
   d. Pyridoxine

5. What kind of vitamins are readily excreted in urine and not stored in the body?
   a. Fat soluble
   b. Botanical
   c. Water soluble
   d. Cyclical

6. The condition of abnormally high storage levels of vitamins which can lead to toxic symptoms is called what?
   a. Vitamin overdose
   b. Hypervitaminosis
   c. Toxic vitamin syndrome
   d. Excessive supplementation

7. Deficiency of which vitamin causes *glossitis, stomatitis*, diarrhea, and skin lesions?
   a. Thiamin
   b. Niacin
   c. Beta-carotene
   d. Pyridoxine

8. What condition can be caused by taking niacin with cerivastatin or red yeast rice?
   a. Rhabdomyolysis
   b. Anemia
   c. Angiomyolipoma
   d. Bartter syndrome

9. Which of the following is not a major form of vitamin C?
   a. Citric ascorbate
   b. Ascorbic acid
   c. Calcium ascorbate
   d. Sodium ascorbate

10. What is the best natural source of vitamin D?
    a. Milk
    b. Whole-grain bread
    c. Sunshine
    d. Cereals

11. If giving B_1 (thiamine) to alcoholics or thiamine-deficient persons, what must be given along with the B_1 in order to prevent Wernicke's encephalopathy?
    a. Magnesium
    b. Saline solution
    c. Potassium
    d. Glucose

12. What over-the-counter drug should be avoided for patients with kidney and liver diseases, stomach ulcers, or bleeding disorders?
    a. Antacids
    b. Cough syrup
    c. Ibuprofen
    d. Antihistamines

13. Which conditions have an absolute contraindication for cannabis use?
    a. Acute psychosis or unstable mental illness
    b. Diabetes and hypoglycemia
    c. Cancer and leukemia
    d. Epilepsy and other seizure disorders